Sickle Cell Disease
Sickle Cell Trait

The Triumphant Struggle of One Man

EZEKIEL SANDY

iUniverse, Inc.
Bloomington

Sickle Cell Disease / Sickle Cell Trait
The Triumphant Struggle of One Man

iUniverse books may be ordered through booksellers or by contacting:

iUniverse
1663 Liberty Drive
Bloomington, IN 47403
www.iuniverse.com
1-800-Authors (1-800-288-4677)

Because of the dynamic nature of the Internet, any web addresses or links contained in this book may have changed since publication and may no longer be valid. The views expressed in this work are solely those of the author and do not necessarily reflect the views of the publisher, and the publisher hereby disclaims any responsibility for them.

Any people depicted in stock imagery provided by Thinkstock are models, and such images are being used for illustrative purposes only.
Certain stock imagery © Thinkstock.

Diet/Exercise Regimens. You should not undertake any diet/exercise regimen recommended in this book before consulting your personal physician. Neither the author nor the publisher shall be responsible or liable for any loss or damage allegedly arising as a consequence of your use or application of any information or suggestions contained in this book.

Medical Advice. The information, ideas, and suggestions in this book are not intended as a substitute for professional medical advice. Before following any suggestions contained in this book, you should consult your personal physician. Neither the author nor the publisher shall be liable or responsible for any loss or damage allegedly arising as a consequence of your use or application of any information or suggestions in this book.

ISBN: 978-1-4759-8615-0 (sc)
ISBN: 978-1-4759-8616-7 (ebk)

Printed in the United States of America

Library of Congress Control Number: 2013907037

iUniverse rev. date: 04/21/2013

Dedicated to those who currently struggle with this disease.

Contents

PART ONE
INTRODUCTION

Putting Things Together

During the last few weeks it has been in my thoughts to write this book on sickle cell disease and sickle cell trait. On the sixteenth day of November, 2007 I was on a bus trip to Washington, DC to attend a march on hate crime. You see, one of my sons, Michael, was killed in Brooklyn, New York and it was a hate crime. I was going there to gain a better understanding about hate crimes.

While on this bus trip to Washington, D.C., I met this lovely lady who was sitting across from me. We struck up a conversation when she offered me a piece of chicken and I said, "No thank you, I don't eat meat."

She then asked me if I was a vegetarian. I said, "No."

One thing led to another and she eventually wanted to find out how much I knew about nutrition and how I got started. By the time I was finished telling her about my health issues with sickle cell she said to me, "You have to write this book."

I told her that for years many people had been advising me to write a book on health and I kept telling them that I was not in the writing business. She told me to pray about it. She also said to me, "I am sorry for your loss; we don't have the answer for everything but God will bring you through this and you will see your son again."

My name is Ezekiel Jeremiah Sandy and this is my story. It is a story about a young man who suffered with this debilitating disease called Sickle Cell Anemia/Sickle Cell Trait and triumphed over it. The information given in this book could be used for all acute diseases of the body.

In 1966, I worked for the US Navy and every few months I went to the hospital for a medical check-up and each time I failed the medical because there was a problem with my blood and urine. I was not given a diagnosis then. I understand that I had been sick off and on as a child and I was told that I was hospitalized for six months on one occasion. In my early years the only diseases I knew or heard of were chicken pox, measles, malaria, typhoid fever and lumbago. I knew nothing about sickle cell or sickle cell trait. As far as I knew, none of my kinfolks had sickle cell. Some say that it appears in the second or fourth generation.

In 1968, I was discharged from the Navy because the base was being closed. I drifted around for a while and ended up at a naval base in Barbados. While I was there I met a medical doctor from the University of London named Ivan Beckles, who was also an herbal practitioner. His wife was a nurse at the local hospital in Barbados. I was quite privileged to spend six weeks with him. Dr. Beckles also had an office on the Island of St. Lucia. One week he went to St. Lucia to visit his patients and I had the opportunity to run the office. I dressed wounds and mixed herbs for the few days I was there in his office.

Time was running out for me; deep in the back of my mind I knew something was wrong with me. I kept telling myself that everything was fine. Two years later I began working again as a welder and rigger building water tanks and performed rig work on three-story building. One morning at about four o'clock I awoke and was wet all over, cold sweating, trembling and shaking. I was also very weak. I changed into dry clothes and went back to bed. Many things went through my mind. At that time I was living with a family member whose name was Elvira Christian. I did not want to wake her so early in the morning so I stayed in bed until six o'clock. I called for a cab to take me to work and when I got to my destination and tried to get out of the cab, my legs were very weak; I was barely able to walk so I held on to the fence while I walked to keep me from falling. I was able to get to the job site without collapsing and I lay on a bench until the rest of the crew arrived.

As soon as the crew saw me, one of them said, "Zeke, you don't look good; do you want to go to the hospital?"

I said, "No."

Tom, the foreman on the job site, remarked that I was turning blue then he said he was going to get coffee and inquired whether any one wanted anything. For some reason I asked him to get me a quart of milk. I was not a milk drinker because I did not like it but at that moment I had the urge for milk.

Let me back up here a little. All through this ordeal, my whole body was itching; I had joint pains, headache and nausea.

Tom said, "Zeke, I don't want you to die on the job; get in the jeep."

Carl and Tom helped me in the jeep. All I wanted to do was sleep but Tom kept saying, "Don't go to sleep; we are almost there."

It was a twenty-minute drive from the job site. When we arrived and pulled up at the emergency entrance, a couple of the EMS guys placed me on a stretcher and took me to the emergency room and Tom called a doctor to take a look at me. It took a few minutes before the doctor could see me. However, as soon as he laid eyes on me he said, "This man is poisoned."

I was already blue. They had to work fast to pump my stomach and fill me up with injections and IV in my system. I don't remember how long it took but the doctor asked whose idea it was for me to drink milk. He said that the milk I drank saved my life because it slowed down the poison but within another day I would have died. I spent four days in intensive care and another few days in a regular ward before I was discharged from the hospital.

After a few weeks I went back to work; everyone was glad to see me because we were a team. I was the main welder on the job and Carl and I were close. We worked well on heights together. Bill's wife had divorced him and, as a result, he drank a lot of whiskey. He was therefore unstable so Carl and I depended on each other's ability when we worked on heights.

I was in the tank building many years before. For example, in 1957 a movie called Swiss Family Robinson was filmed in the Caribbean. This is the original version in which John Mills starred. The movie company rented the welding equipment and I was sent along with the equipment. They paid me fifty dollars a day and the welding equipment. My job was to make sure that the cages holding live sharks were secure and safe. They were large steel cages measuring approximately twenty to thirty feet and a guy called Cecile who weighed about 300 pounds had to go into these cages to wrestle with these sharks. So they depended on me to make sure that these cages were welded strong so that there were no accidents. There was a raft about a mile from the shore and I would swim alongside it for safety. I was a very good swimmer back in those days.

The job of tank building had almost come to an end and one day while we were finishing up Carl received a letter from a company in Alaska offering him a job to work on a barge. He asked me if I was interested. Apparently the pay was very good. I told him I would think about it because my health was not the best. A few days before we were finished I got hurt on my left hand and was rushed back to the same hospital. The young doctor who was about to stitch the wound inquired whether I wanted to be put to sleep.

I said, "No, just go ahead and do it."

He then said to me, "We need young men like you in Vietnam."

I informed him about my health problems and warned that I would be no good to them because I was ill very often. The doctor wanted to examine my medical records to determine what the problem was. At that time they were trying to get recruits to send to Vietnam.

The job finally ended. We did not accept the job in Alaska. Carl went diving for wreckage off the island of St. John's and Bill went back to Texas. I cannot say where Tom went but he was also from Texas.

I knew I had a health issue and I did not know how to deal with it. I used to wake up at nights with my clothes soaked. I would have these dreams at night that I was falling off those tanks and after a while I became fearful of heights, even to this present time. The highest I have ever been was when my son, the late Michael and I were in Palm Springs, California and we took the tramcar to the top of the San Jacinto Mountain. I was usually faced with the questions: Where did this disease come from? What caused it? When I could not find the answer I started to drink

Canadian Club (a brand of whiskey which was referred to as CC) and Coca Cola.

Then one day my Aunt said to me, "You don't look too good, why don't you go and stay with my sister. It would be good for the kids. You never met them; you will be a good big brother to them."

The year was 1972. I had been in Puerto Rico, St. John and St. Thomas in the U.S. Virgin Islands. I returned to my new home in East Farmingdale where my aunt and cousins were living. Bobby had returned from being stationed in Germany during Vietnam War; he was one of the Green Berets who returned home from duty. And John had just gotten back from Vietnam. It was a great time for us to come together as a family and get to know each other while spending quality time together.

All during these times I had good days and bad days regarding my health. The bad days outnumbered the good. It was nice to meet this side of the family so that this historic relationship that I had been missing is fulfilled.

There were others cousins: Bernice, Arlene, Sonny, Jackie and Bertwin. I was the stranger. They heard a lot about me from their mother Rehenia but they never met me until the summer of 1972. They all were waiting at the house to see this man their mother talked so much about. I was 5'6" tall, weighed 146 pounds and looked like I had a few months to live. Arlene fell in love the first time she saw me. They had lots of food—colored greens, black-eyed peas, fried chicken. Granny brought some pig-feet soup. Now, pork was one meat I did not eat. I remember when I was a little boy, my mother used to cook pork. In those days we did not own a refrigerator so when meat was cooked any leftover was covered in a pot and heated and used the following day. When pork was cooked and left overnight the oil used to turn into hard cream. By merely looking at it made me sick to my stomach. So when Granny brought me the pig-feet soup, I became nauseous.

When Bernice got home from school she took one look at me and ran downstairs. She was much older and matured as a fine young lady. She was studying to become a nurse. At the time Aunt Gwenie had lost her husband. She was still going through the effects of losing a loved one so my being there took some of the heavy load off her. Before her husband died he operated a cleaning business and earned his living cleaning offices. However, now the kids and I would assist Aunt Gwenie to clean these offices at nights. My funds were running low and, as a result, I had to find something to do. I would get the newspapers and search for a job. I did not have a car and there was only one in the family and that was a 1970 Ford Maverick.

One Sunday while I was looking in the employment section, I saw a few jobs listed and I selected the one closest to where I lived at that time, which was in East Farmingdale. The job was on Straight Path, Wyandanch. I was there very early and the boss came in at eight o'clock. His name was Marvin. I introduced myself and he asked me if I could do body and fender repair.

I said, "Yes." He then showed me a few cars and asked me if I could fix them and I again said, "Yes."

Despite the fact that I had not done bodywork for quite a while. I had no tools of my own so he provided me with some. I was a bit scared that I would become ill on the job the first day. However, during the course of the day Marvin called the newspaper and cancelled the advertisement because he thought he had found the right man for the job. Marvin was interested to know where I learned to produce such high-quality work at such a fast pace. I was producing and I was not taking any breaks as the other workers. My greatest concern was not being able to last out the week without any setbacks. Luck was in my favor.

I handed over my first paycheck to Arlene to take what she wanted. After all, she was doing my laundry and providing me with meals every day. She surprised me by taking only ten dollars for personal things. Although I sometimes gave money to the rest of the kids for their daily lunch or for books when they needed that, I also saved some money to purchase a car of my own.

One weekend while we were chillin' out, John said, "Let me take you to see my father-in-law in Copiague."

When we got there he introduced me. We had a conversation with father-in-law concerning his wonderful time working with the sanitation department. While there, the father said, "Let's take a walk in the backyard."

There was this 1952 Chevy pickup; it was old, rusty and covered with leaves. As always, my taste for old cars was a gem. My specialty is restoring them. I asked John if his father-in-law would sell me the pickup. The father thought about it for a while then gave me a twenty-five dollar price tag I could not refuse. I paid him the money and he helped me tow the truck over to my aunt's house. I worked on the truck in the afternoons when I got home from work. One day during the winter months; it was about 30 degrees and snowflakes were falling. I was underneath the truck fixing the brakes wearing a t-shirt and a light summer jacket.

Arlene came out running towards the truck yelling, "You know that you are sick and you are out there in the cold!"

I never saw Arlene this way. I apologized for my actions. It took months for me to get back on good terms with her, but the rest was history. The restoration was a success.

I felt that I needed to be honest with my employer. I had not told him of my ill health. He started cooking lunch on the job for me: steak, potatoes, white bread and soda. I was his number one boy. I thought about, on a daily basis, if I should tell my employer that I have an illness because I always tried to be straightforward with others. One day after work I approached him and asked to speak to him.

He wanted to know if I was going to quit the job; he was relieved when I said, "No." He also informed me that he paid me more than the other workers.

I said to him, "I have some heath problems and when I become ill and I don't show up for work, you know that I am confined to bed."

He wanted to know if there was anything he could do to assist when I got sick; he also wanted to know the nature of my illness. I told him about the pains that I went through and that it was something with my blood. I did not want to go into any further details.

I continued working at the job repairing cars. I also finished fixing the brakes on the Chevy; they were all frozen up as a result of the years the pickup was parked there without being used. I gave it a new interior and a paint job and as soon as I was finished with it, my boss's brother who owned the gas station expressed an interest in it and I sold it to him at a fair price. So I was right back where I started, with no wheels.

My cousin John bought a 1966 Chevy Lamans and we started to hang out at the pubs in the Bronx and Harlem. Before you knew it, I began drinking a whole lot. In those days many of the brothers would be strung out on dope and some of them even overdosed on the stuff. It was all around in the clubs. I was always against taking drugs but I was drinking alcohol. Now, the music that was played in the clubs at that time was by

James Brown, Otis Redding, The Chambers Brothers, Smokey Robinson, Aretha Franklin and many others. We usually danced all night and John would drop me off and then I would get up at seven o'clock to go to work. My behavior started to affect Arlene. At these crazy hours we were getting in we used to pick up a hamburger on the way home for the dog so he would not bark.

I would take off my shoes and tiptoe into the house but the wooden floor will still creak and she would get up and say, "I am not sleeping. Why are you coming in so late?"

She would always keep a plate of food under the bed for me so no one would get up during night and eat it. It didn't matter how much I told her I was fine she would always be up when I got in.

After a while I began experiencing pounding headaches and then I would throw up. I would get very weak and my feet would become swollen. I had no insurance and a little money saved so I refused to go to the doctor. I recalled some of the things that were given to us as children when we were sick; things like castor oil and also some of the spices. There was a wide-leaf plant that was used for headaches. I do not know the name of it but when any one of my siblings got a headache, my mother would wrap it around the head with a piece of cloth and this eased the pain. These headaches used to cripple every organ in my body. They left me helpless for days before I could regain my strength. Everyone was nagging me about my drinking and partying with the ladies. I promised to stop the drinking for a while and I did, until the guys on the job started rolling dice on Friday afternoons after work; and then came the beers, the sodas and the girls.

One Friday, Bobby picked me up from work and on our way home he informed me that we had to move. My Aunt put us all to sit down and told us that the state was buying up the lands where we lived. Everyone broke down in tears. This was a very close family. Now, the place that I am speaking about is East Farmingdale. It used to be the Fairchild Facility where planes were rebuilt and parts manufactured. There was a short runway and the authorities bought out the rest of the property with the intention to extend the runway. However, the extension never materialized. Nowadays it is referred to as the million-dollar airport.

Searching for Home

I had to find somewhere to live so I began searching for a place. In the meantime, I asked Marvin, my boss, if he knew anyone who wanted to rent a room to a single man. A few days later a gentleman came into the shop for some minor work to be done on his car. Marvin asked him if he knew anyone who had a room to rent as one of his employees was interested. He also assured him that I was a very nice young man, hardworking and came from a good family.

Marvin called me and introduced me to Mr. Lou. He agreed that I seemed nice and handed me the address. Because I did not have a ride, he offered to take me. He lived a mere five minutes from the job so it was within walking distance. When he reached the house he called out to his wife, Mrs. D. She was beautiful and well spoken. She was from St. Louis and he was from Pensacola, Florida. It was quite a lovely two-story house. There was a living room, kitchen, bedroom and dining room downstairs with beautifully tiled floors. So instead of a one room, I had the entire downstairs with a large backyard. I was so excited I could not wait to move in. I moved that weekend because I did not have much, just my clothes and a few other things.

Mrs. D. seemed friendly but I suspected that she was lonely. During my second week there, Mrs. D. was visited by a girlfriend and she did not hesitate to inform her about this nice man who was living downstairs. This lady, Mrs. D's girlfriend, would go on to play a tremendous role in my life down the road, as it relates to my health problems.

As I mentioned earlier, I began to experience quite a lot of pains. I worked hard, returned home and slept and there were times when I went to bed without eating. Sometimes I got up at two o'clock in the morning and walked to the club, which was not too far from where I lived. Sam, the couple's dog, became a good friend. Every time I got ready to go somewhere Sam was ready to tag along. He used to sit outside the club and wait for me; he was a reliable companion. Sometimes when I returned home Mr. Lou would just be getting home drunk and he would argue with his wife. One night I listened in on the conversation and found out that he had a girlfriend. He frequently came home drunk and abused his wife.

One cold, rainy Saturday evening looking through the window, I saw Mr. Lou slumped over on the stoop. He would have frozen to death if I had not arrived at that time. This was a big guy about two hundred and fifty pounds. I lifted him up and brought him into the house. I changed his clothes and put some dry clothes on him. Later that evening he started to abuse his wife. I was in no shape to stop him. I kept yelling at him, banging on the ceiling and pleading with him to stop hurting her. She finally broke free and ran into the woods on that cold, rainy evening. I went looking for her a little later and found her huddled up under some bushes. I heard him yelling out her name but I was able to get her into the house through the back.

When her girlfriend visited that weekend and saw her face and body all bruised, the girlfriend tried to find out what happened, but Mrs. D. would not say. When I was asked about her, I informed her that the husband was abusing her. The girlfriend was very angry with him. I, myself, never like men who beat women. This turns me away from them.

The girlfriend and I were finally introduced to each other. I will call her Re. She kept coming out on the weekends and always inquired about me. She wanted to know if I had any visitors and Pat told her that my cousin comes to see me sometimes. Re kept visiting there because she knew I was hurting. I was in pain most of the time; I did not have any insurance and the little money I saved so far was to purchase a car so that I could move around on those cold days.

In the meantime something was brewing on at the job. As I said earlier, the guys started to roll dice in the evenings; the work was not getting done as fast as it used to and they depended on me to carry the load, but my health was worsening.

The police department was notified about the gambling that was taking place on the premises. All those company boys were coming over when they heard about the big dice games going on at this location. The employer forgot all about the business; he was also involved in the gambling. As time went by some of the others brought in cocaine and pot. Meanwhile, the law enforcement was keeping an eye on things. Finally, they swooped down on the place. They had enough evidence to put everyone who was involved in the dice game in jail then shut down the establishment.

Once again I was out of a job. The owner of one of the companies that brought us jobs took a liking to me and I mentioned to him that I needed a car since I sold the restored gem for three hundred and fifty dollars. He promised that he would let me know if he saw anything suitable at the auction. A few months went by before I got a call asking me to come and take a look at something that he had found. I got a ride on the weekend to see the car; it was at the back of his office. My eyes lit up when I saw this beauty. It was a four-speed 1969 Pontiac GTO, maroon with black vinyl top and chrome wheels. I inquired about price and was told that it was twenty-five hundred dollars. It took me a few months to gather the money but I bought the car and I had quite a long relationship with it.

I found another job on Long Island Avenue at a BP gas station. Kenny, the owner, was interested in finding someone to do some bodywork on cars. He tested my skills and he liked what he saw. I worked there for about a year and we got to know each other quite well. He would invite me to his home to have a few beers and talk about cars. We put together an Oldsmobile and we would street race and take it to the track.

Although his car was running in the eighths and my GTO was running in the fourteenths, I used to beat him on the streets. We continued working together, however, there was not sufficient work coming in. Sometimes for two or three days there was nothing for me to do. I had a car payment, rent to pay and food to buy so I had to find something else to do. In the meanwhile, I did odd jobs by repairing vehicles for friends who were involved in fender benders. I repaired the vehicles at their residences.

My friend Pete would visit me on weekends. He would bring some of his friends to see my car and tell them how fast it could go in a quarter mile. On one of Re's visit she asked Mrs. D. to find out whether I wanted to go to Nassau County Medical Center because free medical check-ups were given there. I thought she just wanted to get me into Nassau County because it sounded too unreal that a hospital would provide free medical check-ups. I wondered to myself why this woman was doing all this for me when she did not even know me. Now I understand that Re was a smart lady who graduated from one of the finest colleges that a middle class family could send their children to in that era, Tuskegee University, Alabama.

One day Re inquired from Mrs. D. how the guy downstairs was doing. She told her that I had all the women in the land out at my apartment. Now mind you, these were some of the girls from the club who would come over when I hadn't shown up; then one thing led to something else. It was a cool thing in those days when a young man had his own place and drove a nice car. Women liked that; it showed that the man had some ambition. Before you knew it I was running the streets with all those ladies. I would have one hour sleep a day and would be up and ready to hit the road.

I received a call from Mrs. D. one day informing me that the guy from Long Island Avenue wanted me to come back to work. I was happy to hear this bit of news because in those days good help was hard to find. I started working again. Once again, everything was going fine. I began to have a few dollars in my pocket, however, problems flared up at the house that I rented. The abuse resumed.

I got home one evening and Mr. Lou said Mrs. D. was in the hospital and he needed me to go with him but first we had to stop to pick up some lingerie for her. He did not know her size so I had to figure that out. She was small boned, slim, about five feet seven inches tall and weighed about 102 pounds. We stopped off at Macy's to purchase the items. I guess it was a good time to talk to him.

I said to him, "Mr. Lou, what you are doing is not good. The couple of years I have been living there I haven't seen Mrs. D. do anything wrong. She keeps a clean home, she is a good cook, she does not hang out like other women; she is a good housewife."

All he said, "She makes me mad."

I replied, "That still does not give you the right to hit her." I reminded him that the last time he was drunk she could have left him in the snow and rain to freeze, but she did not. I was in for a big shock.

On our way back he said, "I have to make a pit stop."

We got off the highway, drove through the neighborhood and then came to a dead-end street and he asked me to give him a minute. I was in the car for about half an hour. It was quite cold in the car. Finally, he called out to me and asked me to come into the house. Guess what? He had another woman who gave birth to a seven-pound baby.

I was shocked, as she was nothing like what he had at home from what I could see. He asked me not to tell his wife. I felt hurt. Anyway, we left soon after; he could not stay as long as he wanted because he was a truck driver and he had to leave at two o'clock in the morning to go to work. I never told his wife. His mother would come up in the summer to visit him and he would take her to see her grandson.

I began searching for another place because I wanted to move out. Due to my health condition it was important for me to find a new place because there was too much going on in my surroundings. However, I got to thinking about where should I move to or whether I should move at all. After all, I had an okay job and I did not have to travel too far to get there. I think I am getting ahead of myself.

One day Pete said to me, "I want to buy your car; I have been saving up for it."

I told him that my GTO was not for sale but he offered me twenty-five hundred dollars for it. I agreed to sell there and then but I asked him for a few weeks to get something taken off the vehicle. Now, two thousand was put aside for my burial; I wanted a decent burial.

More bad news, my landlord's wife got out of the hospital and was doing okay but after a while the abuse started again. One day when he returned from work she was not at home. She had gone back to her hometown, St. Louis. He went down there to get her but the cops were waiting on him because he had a gun, which he intended to use to threaten her family. When he found out that the police were there, he turned back. She never came back to him.

PART TWO
THE DIAGNOSIS

The News You Don't Want to Hear

For someone who was so ill, I was living an inadequate lifestyle. I was partying and not getting enough rest. I took sick once more and took Advil for the pain. I started passing blood in my urine. I was bleeding quite a lot. The next morning, as sick as I was, I drove myself to Nassau County Medical Center. When I got to the emergency room they thought I had a cut until I informed them that I was bleeding when I passed urine. They took blood and urine samples and managed to stop the bleeding by administering different kinds of medication. They discharged me without letting me know what was wrong but they gave me certain instructions such as no drinking of alcohol and to cut back on my salt intake.

A few days later I was asked to come to a specific clinic at the hospital to see a particular doctor. When I arrived, the clinic was filled with mothers, babies and young teens. I inquired from the receptionist whether I was in the right clinic.

She asked for my name, she looked up a sheet and she said, "Yes, this is the right clinic." She asked whether I was the patient and I said yes.

Finally my name was called. I was a bit nervous but she pointed to the room in which I should go. I entered and there was a male doctor. Now, I had butterflies in my stomach because I did not know what the diagnosis would be.

He said to me, "Mr. Ezeke, you have some serious problems."

He asked me all these crazy questions about whether my family had a history of any blood disorder.

I asked what that had to do with me and he said, "You have a blood disorder that we would like to trace to see which of the family, whether it was your grandparents or parents."

I informed him years ago when I was working in the Navy, I was told that something was wrong with my blood.

He then said, "You have to come here to this clinic twice a week for more tests."

Then I asked, "Why do I have to?"

His response, "You have sickle cell disease or sickle cell trait so you have to come to the clinic." He continued. "All those kids out there have the disease. This is a special clinic; if you don't come for the treatment you will die."

He handed me literature to read.

I stumbled back to the parking lot and got into my car. I sat there for about half an hour, dazed and stunned at the news I just received. I thought of the images of all those children and teenagers in all pitiful forms. I drove home that day and did not remember if it was hot or cold or raining. I walked into the house, went into my bedroom, locked the door and did not eat or sleep for about three days.

I just lay in bed asking myself, "What is sick in the cell? What is a trait sick in the cell?"

If you asked me about doing bodywork on cars and painting them or mixing colors or being on top of tanks or ten-story buildings or let's go further, if you asked me what time of the day it is, so long as the sun is shining I could tell you these things. I have been taught these things from a child. I came from a farming background and the ocean floor. I could tell about the soil and plants. These are the things I knew about but "sick in the cell" (that is what I referred to it), I didn't know about that.

This was 1974; after twenty years I finally found out what I was suffering from and that I would die if I do not take care of it. This is when I said to myself, "I'm a dead man walking."

In those three days I kept getting flashbacks about a Jewish man who had escaped along with his daughter from the concentration camp. This man had accumulated a lot of wealth in a short space of time and he subsequently became very ill. He asked his daughter to charter a plane, find the best doctor and bring him back to treat her father and restore him to good health. The daughter left for London. In those days, anything that came out of Oxford University was top of the line; all the great minds came out of the British Empire.

The daughter returned with a doctor; he had his medical bag, which he held on to as though it contained gold. All his medical tools, his medical books and other apparatuses were in that bag. The patient was on the third floor of his stone mansion; we call them brownstone. The daughter introduced the doctor to her father. The doctor teamed up with the staff to study the nature and the cause of the illness. However, the patient was dead in thirty days. The doctor claimed that he performed everything that medical science had taught him.

The reason I bring up this subject is because when I was a young boy we were told that poor, sick people die because they do not have the money to pay the doctor; only rich people live when they get sick because they could afford to pay the doctors. I kept asking myself, this man had money, so why did he die?

Trust Your Doctors?

Now Re played a major role in my struggle with this acute disease. She was recently divorced and had three wonderful sons. As a result of her efforts I attended the clinic twice a week. They would put me in something like a large washing machine. I did not know what they were doing but they were the experts and I trusted them. Then there were days I was injected with this blue liquid; I was also kept in an upright position. I was told they had to kill the body for a second. I remember one day I kept looking at the clock to see what time I had died. When I woke I usually could not see; I would actually lose my sight. Re would pick me up and take me to her house.

The kids would say, "Here comes the blind man!"

It would take days before I regained my sight fully. These were horrible and frustrating ordeals, especially when I was in a strange environment.

I have seen many blind people in my time but I will only mention two of them who amazed me. There was a blind man who worked at the Federal Building in Richmond, Virginia. He was a cashier at the cafeteria. This man impressed me. It did not matter what bill you gave him, he always gave you the correct change. He was just amazing. Just the past Thanksgiving I inquired about how he was doing and I was told that he got hit while crossing the street and died.

The other person is Betty who was eighty-six years old. Her husband had died and she lived alone and did everything for herself. One week there was an announcement on the radio about a storm that was going to hit her area very hard. I knew that the only station she listened to was the Boston Radio Station. I tried calling her but she did not answer the phone. I drove about forty miles; it was very windy, branches were falling and the power had gone out. I was hoping the constable in the area would have checked on her but they were busy.

Now, she lived in a small house above the lake; the ocean flowed into the lake and the water could rise and reach the foundation of her house. When I got there the water was up to the house. Luckily no great damage was done; a branch had fallen on the house. Apparently the cat had knocked the phone off the hook and since it was a long cord she could not find the phone. When I found her she was laying on the floor and she had been there for a few days, very much afraid. She said when she heard the crashing wave hit against the wall and the branch fall on the house she thought it was all over for her.

Those were the two blind people I admired.

I share those stories because it is a horrible experience when you don't have your sight. Sometimes when I temporarily lost my sight during those treatments, I felt so hopeless but nonetheless, I learned to depend on my sense of smell, my hearing, and my sense of touch. One of the hardest things for me was to listen to a grasshopper leap from one place to another and tell where it landed. I had to relearn things just in case I became permanently blind.

Because of all these trips I had to make to the clinic, it became necessary for me to move closer. I was living in Suffolk County and to get to the hospital was difficult without personal transport so I once again began searching for a room. I was so used to my independence and also, I needed my space in those times of great physical pain.

As time went by, everything seemed to get harder and harder. I threw my hands up in the air on several occasions, ready to give up but Re kept telling me that things would change. My biggest test was at the onset of the pain. Sometimes I felt as though I was going insane.

I finally got a room in Uniondale with an elderly couple, very nice people. My rent was twenty-five dollars a week. I did not disclose my health problems to them. As long as I did not drink, smoke and curse, they did not mind.

I moved into this room and got settled in. I took the bus to get to the clinic for my treatment. When I received these treatments I used to be ill for a week or two. It seemed to me that I was one of their special patients who they were experimenting on because despite all these treatments I was not getting any better. Sometimes I forced myself to visit the clinic and when I complained to the doctors they would say, "Give it time." Or, "If you don't take this medicine you will get worse and even die."

I was frequently depressed. Everything seemed to be closing in on me.

Re did not live too far from me so she would bring me something to eat and she kept encouraging me. On one of my bad days I stayed in bed and during the day the pain intensified and the more I popped painkillers the worse I seem to get. The couple was always up early and for about five days they had not seen me or heard any movement in my room. They used their key to get in because I was not answering their calls. From the stench in the room and when they saw me they thought I was dead until they got closer, heard my groans and saw the pill bottle on the floor. They put me in their car and rushed me to the nearest hospital, which was Hempstead General Hospital.

I went into a semi-coma. I was fortunate to have had my clinic card on me. The hospital immediately contacted the medical center and received instructions from them. Both hospitals worked together to get me out of the state in which I found myself. I was one of the patients who had a microfilm hanging on a chain around my neck and a card to carry at all times just in case anything went wrong with me. The card identified that I was a sickle cell case. When I returned from the hospital my landlord was very upset with me because I did not inform them of my illness. They saved my life that day and I am grateful to them.

One of the things I observed during my illness was that all my party friends disappeared. None of them came to visit me to see if there was anything they could do for me. However, the elderly couple checked in on me twice a day; they would provide me with hot soup and also dinner.

When I offered them extra money they refused; they said, "You are like family."

One day I went to the clinic as was my custom and I was sent to another office. I was terrified as I walked down the corridor to the office because I did not know what to expect. I knocked on the door and entered the room. There was a lady sitting at a desk with my folder in front of her.

She said, "Relax."

Apparently she observed that I was a wreck. She asked me if I was working.

I answered, "When I can, I work to pay my rent but I don't have any great income coming in."

She said, "You have a chronic disease and you need to be on constant medical treatment." She was speaking a language that I did not understand.

I was sent to the SSI Office, in the same county, to apply for social security. They already had my records so they were pretty well informed of my health situation. After weeks and months of what I called interrogation—remember, I did not ask for their help; the hospital recommended me to them for assistance because they thought I was qualified for assistance.

Have you ever tried to get SSI? It was like pulling an infected tooth. After a few months I was turned down and told to go to the social service office. After the experience with the SSI, I was reluctant; after all that running back and forth I was discouraged about approaching another agency but Re was persistent that I should go. I was finally swayed. SSI referred me to Social Service.

When I arrived at the office it was filled with people with all sorts of problems and we were all seeking the same help. As I looked at all the sad faces of those people in the room: mothers with children, addicts, alcoholics; some were possibly freeloaders looking for a free ride; and then there was the expression of desperation on the faces of those who were turned down.

I keep saying to myself, "Get up and leave."

As I looked around this large room some of the children looked as though they were undernourished. It seemed as though whatever disease was affecting them, they had to bring some kind of proof of that. The blind and the lame were also there. It reminded me of some of the clinics I had been to.

Finally, after being there for half the day, my name was called. I walked very slowly to the desk to which I was directed; my stomach in knots. As I got to the desk the officer said, "Good afternoon Mr. Sandy."

I was ready to urinate on myself. I was very nervous. I kept squeezing my legs. She told me to relax. I informed her that I had to go to the bathroom. I finally returned and was more at ease.

Before she could begin the interview I said to her, "Miss, first of all, I do not want any handout. I always work but because of this illness there are days when I cannot and that is why I am here today, seeking assistance."

Before I could finish speaking she stopped me and said, "Mr. Sandy, from what I see from your records we have been withholding from your employer. You are not taking handout; you have been faithfully paying your state tax and when you are in dire straits this is what we are here for, to help you when you are in need." She then said, "Sign here."

My heart skipped a beat. I was so relieved that this had worked out in a positive way for me. She said that my case was fairly straightforward. She inquired whether I had a car and I answered, "Yes."

I was only allowed to use it to go to the doctor, clinic, hospital and to this office. I was given four hundred dollars for rent and food plus an extra twenty dollars for gas and oil. They were very supportive of me. I had their reassurance that they would do everything in their power to help me. They had seen many of these sickle cell cases at their office and many had died. I was very glad for the encouragement. This was a big difference from the SSI.

I received some sad news one day when I returned home from the clinic that the wonderful couple I was living with had to move. They had sold their home because they could not afford to maintain the property; they were moving into a home for seniors in Queens. I had about two weeks to find a place. If I could not find one in time, I could move back to Re's home; but that was my last resort.

After searching in the local newspapers I found a place with a large room about a mile from where I was living. I went there right away, knocked on the door and an elderly man came to the door and said, "Can I help you, sir?"

I informed him that I was there about the advertisement for the room for rent and he asked me to come in. The room was upstairs; I took a look at it. There was a bathroom in the middle and another room across from me, which was already occupied by someone else.

I asked how much and he said, "Forty-five dollars per week." It was quite a convenient location because it was close to three hospitals in any direction. Also, everything was across the street from me.

I went back to let the couple know that I had found a place. They were happy but I was not because they were more than a landlord to me. They asked if I would visit them when I am well; they gave me the address. I must confess that I never went to look for them as I promised, but they were always in my thoughts. Many times when I was sick I sometimes lay in bed and just wished to see someone I knew. During my illness I was always lonely but there was someone always there. I never knew until later on.

The year was 1974. I was living in Nassau County and I continued to battle with my health. I informed Social Service of my new address and they advised me that I just had to explain why I was moving and provide letters from the former landlord and the new landlord and also the new rent I had to pay. The paperwork went through quickly so they could take care of my funds. There was no cost to me at the hospital or the clinic where I went twice a week for treatment.

I informed the new landlord of my health problem. I also let him know that twice a week I must go to the hospital for treatment and I had to take the bus because I couldn't see after these treatments. He offered to take me to the hospital and I told him I didn't want to impose on him. He, however, insisted that he would drive me there, wait on me and bring me back. I would offer him money for gas and he would refuse. He would also knock on my door to see if I was okay and then he would invite me down for breakfast in the mornings.

One morning, we were having breakfast of eggs and toast and he was telling me about his grandson who was about 16 or 17 years old. When I met my landlord, his grandson had a liver transplant and the grandfather took it very hard so he was sympathetic towards me, knowing what his grandson went through. One weekend when his grandson visited he showed me the scars. It seemed as though he was actually cut in half to remove the diseased liver and replace the new one.

Back at the hospital there was no good news, there was no improvement in my condition. They reached a point where they did not know what to do with me; they would have a bunch of specialists sit and discuss my sickle cell case. I was eventually assigned to another clinic on Greenwich Street in Hempstead. I did not know who was my new doctor so as I sat there. I had been to this clinic before with my friend, Re, when she took her children there when they had colds, flu or aches and pains, but I was to learn something new at this clinic. I had visited the clinic a few times before they knew that I had sickle cell. They only found out when my files arrived at their office.

Usually when you are a new patient in a clinic you might be the last patient that the doctor sees, so when my name was called they thought it was a girl so when I stepped into the office and the receptionist saw that a man showed up, she said, "Your name Sandy?"

I said, "Yes."

She said, "Why do you have a girl's name?"

I said, "I have the same trouble all the time. I am used to it."

She asked me to get on the scale, then she wrote down the information; she checked my blood pressure and recorded it and then she said, "The doctor will be with you shortly."

Well, I waited about half an hour then lo and behold this tall, attractive lady walked into the room and closed the door. She wore a doctor's uniform and carried her stethoscope and other things a doctor would normally carry. When the time came to send in the next patient I was stunned for a moment. I did not say anything then she kept staring at me. I must have been in a daze for a few moments then I snapped out of it. She was the first Cushite doctor, what you will call black. She was a pediatrician and this was to be my doctor at the clinic. We will call her Rain. She asked me to undress. Now, initially, I had some difficulty with that but I allowed her to examine me. Finally, I had a doctor with whom I was comfortable.

I inquired about the disease sickle cell and she gave me all the medical terms for sickle cell. Of course, I did not know what she was talking about. I asked her to explain a little more in detail so that I could better understand. Then I told her that I didn't really know what it was. She tried to explain it in the simplest way possible. She said that the white corpuscles invade the red corpuscles and eat them.

It was the first time that any one had really explained this in such a simple way. She showed me on a chart how the reaction took place. There are too many medical terms so I will leave that for the medical experts to explain it to you. Later on in this book I will give you my two cents about it. She also said that she would arrange for some of her colleagues to take a look at me.

I left the clinic up beat; I had finally found someone who I could ask questions and didn't feel I was asking anything out of the way. I was very comfortable with her. She was going to investigate further to see whether there was a cure for this disease. She was only working with children with this disease. It appeared that science did not pay much attention to this disease because it was only dominant in the Cush or black race.

I think there is need for more information, more time and more money from the Federal Government to be put into research as far as sickle cell disease is concerned. The number of children I saw at this clinic was astonishing. I did not know anything about other families and their children. I only knew about me, a young man trying to find the best way how to deal with this disease.

Does Drinking Soothe the Pain When Things Get Bad

It had been months that my new doctor had been searching for new information on this killer disease. In the meanwhile, I had been bored and frustrated because I could not enjoy life as others did; I could not do the work I loved: bodywork on cars. One day while looking through the newspaper I saw an advertisement for a body man in Glen Head, Nassau County. I called the number and a gentleman answered the phone.

I said, "My name is Zeke and I am answering the ad in the newspaper for a body and fender man."

After interviewing me, he said, "You got the job."

He was not surprised who I was because he grew up in South Philadelphia where he worked with some of the toughest street boxers and there were many Cushite brothers with whom he made many friends in the early days in Philadelphia.

I went into work the following day and I met the rest of the crew. I was surprised to be introduced to a young Englishman by the name of Nigel with his deep English accent; I could hardly understand what he was saying. I also met John and Neil; I was very much accepted in the team. There were days when I had to push myself. I used to walk with my lunch and sit with Nigel, trying to learn something about the United Kingdom. I found out that his parents did not approve of him leaving the United Kingdom and moving to the United States and to top it off, he married an American girl. So his relationship with his family was strained. As we got closer I learned that some of the other workers did not like him so I became a close buddy to him. I taught him some of the skills of the trade.

When he was trying to figure out something, I would say, "Why don't you try this?"

I did not know that he was not skilled with the body and fender job but the boss liked him and so did I.

The other guys would go to lunch at the bar and have too much to drink and when they returned to work they could not finish their work. They used to talk about the girls in this bar by the train station. Now, the last thing I wanted to be involved with is bar, club or girls. One Friday one of the guys was having a birthday party at the bar. This was a place where everybody knew everybody and their life stories. They even knew who I was, before I got there. My co-workers insisted that I go with them and I relented. I, however, did not know what to expect.

These people seemed to be stuck in one period of time. Some of them wore eighteenth century cowboy outfits; some of them the twenties farmers' outfits and the jukebox in the corner seemed like the first one that was invented. The older ladies wore long dresses and the younger ones sported cowboy outfits with black and brown cowboy boots. They would put a quarter in the box and the songs being selected were Gene Autry's "Yipee-yi-o, Yipee ai-ay" and others by Patsy Cline, Johnny Cash and George Jones. Those were some of the songs I remembered being played there. There were also one or two songs by the Beetles.

I remember back in the sixties on a U.S. Base in the Caribbean there was a radio station and someone called Val was the night Disk Jockey. He would play all those sad Country and western songs as fast as the requests came in but this was the late seventies and these people had not changed. I looked different from them but that did not stop them from coming over and asking to buy me drinks. I felt like I was the guest of honor that night.

Every time I went to the bar the waitress would say, "Your drink has been paid for."

I sat at the end of the bar and the ladies came over and asked me to dance. I was afraid their husbands or boyfriends would come over and say something to me. I kept looking over my shoulder. I could not dance the kind of dances they were doing, but they seemed to be having a ball.

The girl at the bar, a tall brunette who we will call Gen, she kept smiling at me; she wanted to know if I worked with John and Mike. I told her that I was the new guy on the block.

She said, "Everyone is talking about the darkie."

I said, "I hope it is nothing bad," and she answered in the negative.

She asked whether she would see me again and I told her she would find me at the shop. She promised to come by. Very soon, I had several drinks under my belt. I was told by the doctors drinking was one of the things I should definitely refrain from. I had stopped drinking until that Friday night party. I ignored all the warnings. It became a regular pastime. Every Wednesday to Friday there would be drinking and partying. Sometimes the party would end up at someone's house and the next thing I would be surrounded by all these lovely ladies.

Well, the owner of the company I was working for was having some kind of troubles at home so he had to move out. He found a place in a castle on the north shore somewhere in the Locust Valley Estate, some kind of hundred-room house with its own traffic lights. This house belonged to the owner of the Swiss watch company. There were two partners: one lived in Europe and the other lived in the United States. The castle was so huge that you could be at one end and no one knew if you were at the other end. He only drove Jaguars; he was a single man in his forties or fifties at the time. You should see the ladies he rode with; classy dames. Some of them were French ladies. He used to either drop his car off or Mike would bring it to work and we would sit behind the wheel just to imagine what it would be like to own one. When we opened the trunk there would be all these expensive watches in cases, but we would get them for about thirty dollars a piece.

The partying continued and I had been getting home later. My friend, Re, was getting upset; she would go to where I stayed and asked the landlord if I got home as yet. Cell phones were not yet available; it was easy to make up all kinds of excuses about your whereabouts and knowing her I had to come up with some very creative ones. I used to clean my breath when I got to her place because if she smelled alcohol on my breath she would hit the ceiling. Also, she would always chastise me about other women.

I was in too deep to quit the drinking and the partying. Sometimes I would forget to take my medication and this would go on for days. The booze was actually keeping me numb. Sometimes I didn't feel the pain.

Mike would say to me, "Why don't you go home? You look like hell!"

I remember one day it had rained so much that the shop was flooded. I was called upstairs to take a look at a car; it was a yellow Volkswagen. The guy was told to return the car for repairs on the following day. Instead we got a call that he would not be bringing the car because he had died that night. I mention this because I should have been dead a long time ago. A few people that I had come into contact with were dead. I don't want to spend a lot of time on this subject right now, but I will touch on it sometime later.

I continued to struggle with my health. I would take time off to go to the clinic for my treatment. In 1974, I was waiting for the last result of any progress the doctors had made so I kept calling the office to find out if they had any good news. If you were in my situation, any good news was something to rejoice about. In the meantime the business was getting slow. There was some question about whether Mike could hold on to the shop as there was another company interested in the building to carry on the same type of business. I did not have all the details but we had to be out of there by a certain date. It was sad news because we had become like a family: Mike, John, Nigel, Neil and I. We, however, kept in touch with each other. Every other week we met the old gang at a bar in Glen Head; Mike was not always there.

I received some information that I had to return to the hospital for some more tests after which I had to go to the clinic. I felt good that at last I had some positive results. They kept me in the reception area practically all day. Finally I went into the doctor's office and there were two other doctors present. At the sight of both them, I became very nervous. My heart was beating rapidly; I did not know if I would pass out. In their conversations with me they kept going around in circles until they got to the point and dropped the bomb. I must have turned several colors in that clinic. The end result was that I not only had the sickle cell disease but I also had kidney failure, high blood pressure, some kind of brain tumor and I was given five more years to live. Before I left the hospital they gave me a prescription to see a psychiatrist. I made a right turn and headed out to the car, I got in and sat there for about half an hour to compose myself. I finally started the car and cried all the way home.

I went to Re's home to give her the bad news. She knew my hope was fading but she kept offering words of comfort and saying things will be all right.

The kids were asking, "Mom, is he dying?"

The kids were sad because I was a good stepfather to them. Re insisted that we should get another opinion. She made many phone calls on her job to see other doctors on this matter and she located two doctors and set up appointments with them. They ran several tests to see whether the other doctors are wrong. Well after months, they came up with the same answer: I would not live through the next five years. The only thing that they would prescribe is different kinds of medicines to keep my body functioning and psychiatry to help me cope.

We left the doctor's office that day in despair but Re kept saying while we were on our way home that we would keep looking until we found someone who could find the answer. All I was thinking about was the good times I had in the past. I knew deep down inside that I had lost all hope; I had no answer. With tears streaming down my face, all I could think about was that I had five years in which to achieve everything that I always wanted.

These were the winter months; we got to Re's home that night—she thought I should spend the night because I was in no condition to be alone. It was a bitter cold night; the children were already in their rooms so they all came out of their rooms and we sat at the kitchen table. Re told them what the doctor said. I was in no mood to hold conversations so I went out to the driveway and got into the car and locked the doors.

While they were in the kitchen I thought about how easy it would be to end it all. I took a few of the pills and sat in the passenger seat and went to sleep. As I said, it was a very cold night. From what I understand, with the wind, it was about 25 degrees below zero. About an hour later when they did not see me return to the house they thought I had gone for a walk. They came out and looked up and down the block and could not find me.

Re eventually thought of going to my residence to see if I had gone home but she could not find her car key; she thought she had left it on the table, but luckily she had a spare key in the garage. When she got the key and opened the door she found me slumped over like I was drunk. The kids thought I was dead. They were able to get me back into the house and kept me warm; they also tried to keep me awake. I remembered barely hearing voices far away. There was a roomer upstairs who wanted to know what had happened. Re kept saying nothing. The next morning she told me that I had given them a scare. I informed her that I thought about committing suicide and it was the perfect timing, just take the extra pills and go to sleep; there would be no pain.

I was mentally tired. I had been through too much with this disease and now I was dying slowly, according to the doctors. I had taken a large amount of drugs and injections over the years. There were times I could not lay on my back or sit because of the excruciating pain in those areas of my body. I just felt that I had enough. For the next few weeks they kept a close eye on me to make sure that I did not do anything foolish, but I gave them my word that I would not do it again.

I kept weathering the storm. I moved in with Re which I considered a good thing but I kept my old room because there were days when I preferred to be alone. I referred to them as the sad days. I would spend the time thinking about all the good days that my cousin and I had while living in that old house as one big happy family and one day it all disappeared. Like a leaf that fell from a tree and the wind just blew it.

I would sometimes drive to Glen Head and meet my friend John and go to the bar and listen to those sad country and western songs. Sometimes I would punch in a Chuck Berry then everyone would start jumping to kind of snap me out of that fog that I was in. I never understood why Re stayed around me. She knew about my health problem; she was aware that I could die any day and she still wanted to be with me knowing that there was nothing I could offer her.

I was still hanging out and when the pain started I didn't know who I was. I was always afraid. It was a very scary feeling. I kept looking for answers but no one seemed to have any.

The Doctor Visit That Changed My Life

We were now a few months into a new year, 1975 and I needed to acquire the rest of my burial money. I bought a 1973 Seville for four hundred dollars; I fixed it up and sold it for thirteen hundred dollars to an elderly woman who owned a deli. It was enough for my burial with a few dollars to spare. Time was running out for me; the days and nights were getting shorter. I tried to block thoughts of my mortality out of my mind but at times this was impossible.

One day out of the blue Mike called the house and left a message for me with one of the kids. I did not get the message until a few days later. I found out that Mike had a job as a manager at the body shop of a Chevrolet dealership and he wanted me to come on board. He kept the position open for me because he knew I was a very good worker. When I was well I got in touch with him.

Now, John had a job close to home, he never liked to work far away from his home so he was not thrilled to work any distance from his residence, but he gave me Mike's phone number and I made the phone call. Mike inquired about my health and I told him I was still struggling.

He said he had a job, it was unionized and the guys there were not working so I said to him, "You've got your man." He then shared, "By the way, Neil is here."

I was ecstatic because I had not seen Neil for about a year since we split up from the old Glenway. I was satisfied that we would be a team again.

The department in Mike's charge was making money; other departments were not making their quota so they were skimming from off the top of his quota to cover their inefficiency. Since the body shop was carrying the other departments, the CEO pushed the body shop to produce more revenue. There was a difficulty here since the shop did not receive enough work. Mike tried to solve the problem by encouraging some of his old customers to bring their cars to that body shop for repairs.

I kept working through my coffee breaks, lunch breaks and dinner breaks because Mike knew that I was a hard worker. As long as I was well enough I would push a vast amount of work out. Now, for years I had taken lunch to work. One day, it was very hectic and Mike told me that the coffee truck was out there and I should get something to eat. I told him that I had my lunch. At this time some of the guys had gone to the deli and some them were sitting outside.

I was inside working and one of the guys said to me, "Zeke, you need to take a look at this."

I went across to the car; the paint on the fender did not match. I had my steak sandwich;

I took one bite of it; I could not have gone more than five minutes and when I returned and took up the sandwich, it was filled with worms. I could not understand it. I almost vomited. I used to love beef, especially the lean cuts and well done. I then decided to give up meat; so in the summer of 1975 I stopped eating the meat of animals.

I enjoyed the parties, barbecues and the summer fests but I could no longer enjoy these things because meat was always the center of these activities. It was the second time in my life that I had given up some kind of meat.

When I was a boy my mother would cook pork on some special days. Now, pork was poor people's meat because it was more expensive to own a calf and so, most people reared pigs. Whenever pork was cooked, because we did not own a refrigerator at that time in the fifties, it was left to sit in the pot and by the following morning there would be this hard looking cream at the top. I used to get sick by just looking at it. My mother used to put the meat at the bottom of the dish and covered it with rice so that when I put a spoonful of rice into my mouth, there would be little chunks of pork I would spit out. So from a child I would put up a fight not to eat pork. Eventually I gave up pork because I could not stand the look of it.

One afternoon after work Mike and I were chatting about the old times. He asked, "Have you made any progress with your health?"

I answered, "No."

He then informed me that he knew someone who might be able to help me. "I have a doctor who has been helping me." Then he told me that he had been sick.

I said to him, "Mike, all these years I have known you, worked for you, you never indicated that you were sick."

He then explained that every time he smelled paint he passed out and he was put on medication. It was then I understood why he rarely came down to the body shop floor. We always had to go upstairs to seek advice or obtain information and since we were good workers there was no need for him to keep tabs on us. He promised to speak to the doctor about me. He indicated that it was a Filipino doctor. I was a little upset with him.

I asked him, "How do you know this guy could help me?"

And he said, "Give it a shot."

By this time, I had my share of doctors because despite all that I had been through, they could not help.

He then said, "Stick around. I will introduce you to him." He probably realized that I was upset because he barked at me, "You are going to die, nigger."

Let us pause for a moment because I want to inject something. Many times during a struggle in life a window may be opened to you and most times you will turn it down. In my case, Mike as a friend and employer stretched out his hand to me and I did not appreciate it but by using the "N" word and a few other things caused me to act or motivated me to do something. By the time the doctor got there I was still angry because when I shook his hand I was still shaking. He said to me, "I heard you are a good auto body worker." I responded, "I don't know how good I am, but I try." He asked whether I had worked on his car and I said, "No, one of the other guys did." He gave me the address of his office on Jericho Turnpike in Syosset next to the hospital. I called the following day and made an appointment, which was in the next thirty days. Little did I know that something was about to happen that would shift the puzzle to another direction in my life.

By this time I was engaged to Re. We had our ups and down in our relationship. She wanted me to move in permanently but I was reluctant. I was so used to living alone and there were times when I was in the bottom of the barrel and wanted to be on my own. One of the things that were getting bad was the headaches. They would get worse when they came and lasted longer. In between I would visit one of the doctors who would give me medication for the headaches. Now, the medication was not working but he advised me to double up on it, but then I would get very weak and sometimes helpless. My eyesight would get blurry and I would see shadows. I guess this was as a result of the brain tumor. I would have given anything to stop those headaches.

Meanwhile, I was hoping that someone would cancel his appointment so that my appointment could be brought forward. Sometimes I would take a few drinks and hoped that this would stop the pain but it just made me sleep for hours at a time and then I would feel very weak. Sometimes the headaches would disappear but the aftermath would leave me numb. I kept marking the calendar for the date of my appointment.

I saw the Filipino doctor a few times since I made the appointment with his office. He would come by to see Mike and also to get a few touchups on his Lincoln. We did not say much to each other except that I may say "Hi Doc" and he would respond, "See you soon."

The day had finally arrived for my nine o'clock morning appointment. Mike had given me the time off. Since I was working for this company and they had insurance and the shop was unionized, I had to notify the Social Service because they had to give me the okay, a letter in writing and if the doctor or the hospital will be treating me but this was my first visit and from this they were going to send all the paper work to Social Service.

I took the elevator and got off on the second floor of the building, walking slowly to his office. When I opened the door, I thought I was in the wrong office because it was filled with mostly senior citizens. I walked in, went to the receptionist and gave her my name.

She smiled and asked, "You are Sandy?"

I said, "Yes."

"We have you down as 'Miss,'" she said.

I replied, "I'm used to that; I have this problem all the time."

She then said, "My name is Sandy, too."

We chuckled a little then she told me to have a seat. I thought I would be there for about half an hour. I sat in that office and I scanned through all the magazines. I also read some of the articles to see if I could understand any of them. The receptionist went out, got her coffee and came back and I was still sitting there. I was getting impatient and frustrated and then I began having all these negative thoughts. At this time I was not thinking straight. I looked at the clock on the wall; it was now half past ten in the morning and I was still waiting to see the doctor.

Let me take a brief moment here. Now, I know that many of you have had appointments with doctors for specific times but yet you have had to wait for some considerable time before you see the doctor. As I said before, it was a very frustrating situation and I had become quite impatient. However, something great was about to happen; as they say, it is all about timing.

At eleven o'clock, I thrust my hands up in the air and I walked towards the door. As I opened the door and had half of my body in the hallway, the receptionist called my name and said, "The doctor will see you now, Mr. Sandy." I entered the room and closed the door behind me. He then asked me to take a seat and I did.

The doctor shook my hand and he asked, "How is everything at the shop and how is my friend Mike?"

After I responded that Mike was fine, he changed the subject to cars. Now, I had been there since nine o'clock and all he wanted to talk about was his Lincoln and whether we had done a good job on his vehicle when he brought it to the shop for repair. I reassured him that he had nothing to worry about.

The doctor finally asked, "What can I do for you?"

I informed him that I had an appointment. I was somewhat surprised that he did not know about my illness. I explained the problem I was experiencing and then he said Mike had told him some of what he knew about my health woes. Now, I was sitting in his office facing south, looking at the cars running east to west on Jericho Turnpike. He was facing the northern wall with his back towards the south and I sat facing him.

Now and then I would look at the cars on the turnpike going back and forth. The reason I am explaining this to you is because something was about to happen that would bring considerable change to my situation. He questioned me about whether my mother had sickle cell and I said, "As far as I know, no one in my family had this disease or any problem such as mine."

He explained that it was a hereditary problem and my mother had to have it for it to pass on to me. This was the same thing I had been hearing for years; that the disease was hereditary.

PART THREE
THE TRIUMPH

The Bible: A Turning Point

There and then I lost all faith in this doctor because I knew he did not have a solution for my issues. While he was speaking, I lost interest in what he was saying about sickle cell. I was looking at the cars, when suddenly I felt as though a hand had twisted my head from south to east in an upward direction towards the ceiling. My attention was drawn to this large picture on the wall close to the ceiling. It was about four feet long and twenty inches wide displaying all different types of fruits and vegetables. I left his office not remembering much of what he had said to me.

My mind was focused on the picture on the wall. It became a fixed image in my mind all the way home; it was all I could think about. At times I wondered why I had not seen it when I walked in. When I entered his office I saw all his certificates hanging on the wall but I did not see the amazing gift that was there for me. I thought this was destined to work out this way: Mike called me for a job at the car dealership; he introduced me to this doctor from the Philippines and then I waited a month before I could see him. Everything was timed perfectly. This was another lesson I had to learn; that nothing happened before its time.

I owned a white Ford Fairlane 1968 model. I named her Betsy and kept talking to Betsy about what had happened at the doctor's office. I did not mention it to anyone else, not even Re, because they all knew I was on all medication; that doctors had requested me to see a psychiatrist and on top of that, I had tried to commit suicide. I kept this information to myself lest they deemed me insane.

I got home that evening and lay across the bed. Re came by later on and brought me some food. She was eager to know how the doctor's visit had gone but I told her that I couldn't remember everything; all I remembered was that he wanted to know if my mother or anyone in my family had sickle cell disease or sickle cell trait and I told him as far as I knew, no one in my family had it. She kept insisting.

I said, "Why are you asking me all these questions?"

She said, "I want to know."

I then informed her that I wanted to be alone. She asked whether I was coming over later, I said I didn't know and she left.

My mind was on that picture all evening. I didn't sleep well that night. The next morning I got up at four o'clock. I took a ride on the turnpike heading west. Why? Because a few weeks before I went to see the doctor, I was on that same turnpike in that area and I saw a new food store called Buy Rite. It was a new chain-food store that came into the metropolitan area. I got there about half an hour later; it was extremely cold so I kept Betsy running to keep me warm. I parked in a particular way so as not to attract the police that drove back and forth. I did not want it to seem that I was there to hold up the store.

Around half past six, a tractor and trailer pulled on to the compound and went around the back of the store. I tried to get the driver's attention but no one paid any attention to me. Finally, I saw people going into the store and I followed them. The store had opened for early shoppers. I waited until I got some attention then finally this gentleman came up to me and asked whether he could help me and I told him that I had seen some trucks pulling in and going around to the back. He informed me that they brought produce and groceries. I then asked where the produce came from. He inquired why I wanted that information and I told him I merely wanted to know where I could get fresh fruits and vegetables. Unfortunately, he could not provide the information. I looked around for a little while and left. My aim was to find out as much as I could about the picture that I carried around in my head.

I inquired at other stores about foodstuff. I would follow the same pattern: drive early to the food stores and ask the same question about where they obtained their food. Some of the managers did not even know where their food came from. So I had to get to the truck drivers to find out where they were picking up their loads. Finally I was at a particular store and I asked a gentleman where the vegetables came from and he promised to find out. He was not the truck driver; he was just unloading the vegetables from the back. On his return he informed me that the driver picked up his delivery from Hunts Point warehouse. That was all the information he gave me and that was sufficient.

After weeks of chasing trucks early in the morning, my next step was to find out what days the goods were delivered and when was the best time to purchase them. It was a little tricky; I had to learn the system, how to get these different kinds of food.

Let's stop here for a while. I am getting ahead of myself. I know you are waiting for me to tell you what kind of food I used for my illness, sickle cell trait or sickle cell anemia. These diseases affect the body in the same way. The experts may tell you differently but they do not have the disease and experience the pain and some of the deformity that can be caused to the body. Fortunately this book will give you detailed information about the regiment that I used for my illness, however, there is more to it. There will be another book on the subject of health covering those issues in greater detail. So hang in there and be patient. It is all coming to you.

Around this time there was some trouble at my job at the car dealership; the body shop was closed and Mike left. It was said that the body shop was not making money but we all knew differently. Everyone had left but there was news that there was one worker who was very good at his job. I went to pick up my tools and guess what? That section of the body shop was leased to an independent. I went to the office to turn in my uniform to the company and collect my last paycheck.

While I was in the office a gentleman entered the room and the manager said, "Zeke, I want you to meet someone."

We will call this man Bob. After we were introduced Bob asked me to stop by the body shop before I left. I was in the office for about half an hour doing my business when the manager informed me that the new guy who leased the body shop next door wanted to hire me to work for him. I told him he was a good man and thanked him for the recommendation.

Later I went across to the body shop office and Bob was tending to a few customers. While I waited, I looked in the shop and there were some South American Spanish brothers working. One of them asked whether he could help me and I told him I was waiting on the boss. From what I observed while I was waiting, I could tell that they were not experts. They spent a lot of time chatting. Finally, the boss asked me to step into his office. We sat and chatted for a while.

He asked me how I was doing and he informed me that he heard about my health issues then he said, "If you could work with the problem then you are the man I need."

I listened to him and when he was finished I said to him, "I want 'X' amount an hour."

He was taken aback by my request. He then responded, "My guys don't make that amount."

I repeated my demand. He thought about it for a while before he finally agreed.

The following week I started to work for this independent and during the course of the week they all thought I was on some kind of drugs. He said he had not seen anyone worked that fast and producing such quality work and that I was his best man. Now, that created a problem on the job; the rest of the employees would make up stories to tell the boss but I had been used to this kind of behavior in the past. All the other Cushites or the blacks were janitors, cleaners or doing odd jobs. They did not have a trade or a particular skill so it was very nice to see a Cushite who they all could look up to. I did not see Mike for a while; we lost touch with each other. I continued to search for ways to improve my health but every turn I made there were some lessons I had to learn along the way.

The year is 1976. Although it was a promising year for me it also turned out to be a very painful year. I had been doing well for the better part of the spring. One of my doctors at the medical center advised me that it was better to move to where the air was fresher; he felt the fresh air would be good for me.

My relation with Re was getting rocky because she thought I was seeing someone else. Although this was not so at the time, later on in the summer I began using a bank in the Garden City and I met this young Irish girl who was working at the bank. When I went to cash my check. I would say hello but nothing else; then one day I invited her out. However, that week I had one of my attacks, which kept me in bed for about a week. Whenever I had those painful attacks I did not have the desire to eat anything so I went one or two weeks without food. Water or juice usually sustained me. During the course of that week Re called and also visited me to make sure I was okay.

Later that Sunday about two o'clock in the afternoon, I went to use the bathroom in the hallway. As I stepped out of the bathroom and shut the door behind me, I blacked out, fell and rolled down maybe eight to ten steps. I was fortunate that my landlord was at home. His car was always parked in the driveway. I think it was a 1962 Volkswagen; I cannot recall whether it was the Beetle or the Bug but he and the other roomer who was across the hall from me got me into his car and took me to the hospital. Instead of taking me to my regular hospital, which is the County Hospital, he drove me to a hospital in Rockville Center called Mercy.

I was taken to the emergency room and they asked about me and my landlord answered for me.

"He is my tenant and I know he is always sick. I picked him up from the medical hospital in East Meadow a few times."

While I was on the stretcher I could hear sounds as though they were coming from a distance. They checked to see if I had any form of identification on me and found the chain with the microfilm around my neck. The information was put into their system and, bingo, they found out all they needed to know. They knew what medication to put me on and the IV therapy to use.

A few days later I tried to find out where I was and what hospital I was in then the patient who was in the bed next to me said, "They almost lost you."

I asked what he meant.

He said, "They were working on you for quite a while; you were in a pretty bad shape."

I was still very weak and drugged up. I felt very helpless. We exchanged names and he told me that I would be there for a while. I asked how he knew that.

He answered, "When you are on this floor you are usually here for a few weeks. Everyone on this floor has been here for a few months." He continued, "I was told that I was going home soon and I have been here a few months."

I knew then from what he said that I was not going home soon. During our conversation he informed me that he had cancer and they were experimenting with a new treatment. He also told me that a guy had died the night before in the bed I was occupying.

I was on either the second or third floor. There was a large window and I could see the sunrise but I had to get up and look further west to see it set. The reason I needed to see the sun at certain times was that I could tell the time by the position of the sun. During the course of the day there was usually a lot of traffic and I saw many people: families and friends of patients visiting loved ones in the hospital. This lifted my spirits but when the sun went down and the darkness descended on the windows, I became very lonely.

My landlord visited me once while I was at the hospital and I felt very good. I was hoping he would stay a little longer but at his age he did not like to drive at nights since his eyesight was not that good. He wanted to know if I needed anything. I thanked him and I asked him to call my job and inform them that I was in the hospital and he promised to do that for me. The Social Service had sent me my check and I told him to take out his rent but he said he would wait.

One night after the nurses had made their rounds and the lights were dimmed, there was the sound of groans coming from one of the patients who was in pain. I on the other hand was able to withstand the pain without making any noise. I would lay still and absorb the pain but these people could not do it. My friend in the bed next to me said I would get used to what was happening around me, but I did not. I never liked nights at the hospital.

There was also the sound of the elevator door opening and closing and the guy next to me used to say, "Here comes the meat wagon!"

He explained that it was a signal that someone had died. Now, I must confess that his comment sent shivers through me.

He said, "When you hear that sound of the wheels, they are coming for someone."

You would hear that elevator door open and you would hear those wheels of the trolley make this funny squeaking sound coming through the floor to take away someone who did not make it through that night. I used to get as much sleep as I could during the day so that I could stay awake at night.

The nurse would ask, "Why are you not sleeping?"

They would ask me if I wanted a tablet to put me to sleep and I would refuse. I would tell them, "All those shots you have been giving me all day keep me awake."

Re went to see me a couple of times at my place of residence but she got no answer. She went to my job and found out that I was at the hospital but they did not know which hospital I was in. She went back to my place and found the landlord who told her he took me to Mercy Hospital a week ago and I was doing fine. So she came to look for me at the hospital. She did not like what she saw. In her eyes, I was not looking in the best of health. She spent a little while with me and before she left she wanted to know if there was anyone she could contact. She knew little about my cousin; they had all moved away. She knew little about my brother Chris who lived in Harlem at the time. I told her I wanted to get out of there as soon as possible. Before she left, she promised that she would be back to see me.

While I was at the hospital, the staff would come and wheel my friend next to me out of the room and he would be gone for most of the day and when they brought him back he just slept the rest of the day.

One day I said to him, "You are really knocked out today."

He responded that the treatment he was being given knocked him out. He was getting radiation treatment. It was the first time I heard this. It was a new type of cancer treatment. He showed me his body from his chest down to his stomach. There were burns and blisters on his body; blood and puss oozed through the bandage and there was odor coming from his mouth. It left me sick to my stomach. I could not stand staying in the hospital anymore and I decided to leave.

I waited for a busy day to make my move. Now, Monday was usually a busy day; everyone was coming back from weekend trips and days off. Around lunchtime when the traffic was very busy I took the stairs, which were rarely used; everyone took the elevators. I made it down the stairs to the corridor. My next task was to get past the information desk. I made it; I got to the door and I was looking at freedom. It was a busy street and the highway was right there in front of me. There were a few people approaching the door. I hesitated for about a second and one of them stopped to let me out. They started laughing at me because my behind was exposed.

Then someone said, "Do you see that guy standing there with his behind exposed?"

That comment foiled my escape to freedom. The hospital guard brought me back inside and questioned me.

I kept saying, "I want to go home. I want to go home."

The next few days they kept a close watch on me. The nurse would say, "Naughty, naughty. You don't like us. Why do you want to run away?"

I said, "I don't like hospitals."

Her response, "We are only here to make you better so you could go home."

During the next few days my friend's condition began to worsen. The radiation treatments took a lot out of him. He was given extra doses of painkillers for the pain. The next couple of nights I kept an eye on him; he was too weak to go for the radiation treatment the following day. He asked me to go downstairs and get him some ice cream. He opened the drawer next to his bed to get some change but I told him I would handle it. I brought him back a small cup of ice cream; he ate it. It was soft for his mouth because of the mouth sores.

He died within three days. That day I wept bitterly. I stood at that window and prayed. I made a promise to God that if he spared my life I would spend the rest of my days helping people who had health problems.

I do not recall his name; he was of Italian descent from Bellmore, Long Island. He did not have to listen to the death cart coming from the elevator anymore. His death changed something in me. Within a few days I was discharged from the hospital and my landlord picked me up. I spent the next week at home getting my strength back then I got to thinking of all the people who I was close to or getting close to and they had all died.

Howard Hughes had been ill and I heard a lot about the billionaire Howard Hughes, the world's richest man. I don't know what he was thinking while he was ill but I am sure he was getting advice about his wealth and I am sure he must have spent millions for the best kind of treatment to get better, but those doctors failed.

Earlier I told you about a man who sent his daughter to London in search of the best physician. The physician came and did all he knew medically and yet he failed and so will all great doctors because only the Real Healer will heal you when you obey Him completely.

Howard Hughes died in the spring of 1976 before I went into the hospital.

That weekend I went to the laundromat to have my dirty laundry cleaned and while I was there the young lady from the bank came in. I was embarrassed, but I could not hide. If I had seen her coming I would have found some way to avoid her. You see, I do not think I was appropriately dressed.

However, I mustered the courage and said, "Hi."

She said that I looked like a bum. I let her know that I was in the hospital having some tests done, but I did not tell her that I was suffering from sickle cell disease. She then understood why I had not come to the bank for a while. She inquired whether everything was okay with me and I told her I didn't know. I asked whether she lived around the area and found out that she lived on Pierson Avenue. I informed her that I lived on Jerusalem Avenue in Uniondale.

Then she said, "I know the area; I used to work at the bowling alley when I was in high school."

"I am a few blocks from the bowling alley," I responded. I then asked her for her phone number.

She hesitated but I told her I was as harmless as a dove. She wanted to know if I was married and I told her no.

I said to her, "I am here every week about this time maybe we could get something to eat sometime."

She said to me, "We'll see."

By that time my laundry was finished and I said goodbye. I learned something that day: always dress appropriately when you leave your house because you never know who you will run into.

I went back to my room, put the clothes away, got the Sunday Newsday and lay on the bed. While going through the newspaper, I encountered an offer from Doubleday. For the price of one dollar you could select six books from a whole list of different kinds of books and you were also entitled to a free *Bible*. I went through the list and chose six medical books and hoped that they had something on sickle cell or sickle cell trait. I then filled out the coupon with my address and a money order for one dollar. On Monday morning on my way to work, I dropped it in the mailbox.

I had been away from work for a long time. When I got to the job I was expecting the worse but to my surprise they welcomed me back with open arms. I found that my equipment was not in order; someone had used my tools and did not take good care of them. I was very disturbed by this. I cleaned the rest and I had to replace some of them, so it was not a good day for me.

As was expected, there was a backlog of work; most of what was done in my absence was returned so I thought about quitting the job. I reflected on this and decided against it because Bob was kind enough to keep the spot open until my return. I worked through my breaks just to get some of the jobs out.

The boss, Bob, said to me, "I appreciate you hustling to get the jobs out."

I kept working through my lunch hour and the morning and evening breaks just to get the work done. I would hear from the other department that "Zeke is back." I did not know that one man could affect a company in such a way by keeping production up. This weakness showed up whenever I was not there because the other workers did not have the skill or the ability to produce quality work.

I continued to struggle with my health. At nights I would ponder on what I had prayed for while I was at the hospital. One of the things that stayed with me was that I did not have much time to live. I would go to the club and I would drink to drown my sorrows. I used to listen to BB King singing the blues and Ruth Brown, who I knew very well. She used to cook these southern dishes that made you lick your fingers. She used to invite some of the brothers who took care of the car that they went on the road with. I think it was a 1964 or 1966 Lincoln silver grey metallic.

The same thing I was supposed to stay away from, I was indulging in: the women, the partying and the booze. The bottle was my prop. Now, I did not drink at home; I only drank when I went out to party.

It is now the fall of 1976. I was hoping that this new year would bring me some relief. Have you ever been in a position where you felt helpless? I felt there was something to do but I just didn't know what it was. This was how I felt—helpless. The last time I felt like this was when I was a young lad and I was surrounded by critters; I felt paralyzed and could not move. Later in life, I found out that they were there to protect me from further harm.

I continued to hide behind the drink. I was afraid to step outside listening to all the experts who were looking into medical books for the answer and couldn't come up with a cure for my illness. I was just a helpless man with nowhere to turn but the Canadian CC (rum and coke) in a glass at the club and the bars. That was my real medicine; and then when I got wasted I would cry and ask for help and I would promise myself never to take another drink. However, the following week I would do the same thing all over again.

A few weeks after I mailed the coupon to Doubleday, I received a package from the post office. It had finally arrived. I was excited and thrilled. I opened the box without any hesitation. There were the books I picked out and my free *Bible*. I took out the books and searched for anything that could relate to my illness; I spent the time at nights looking through these books to find anything to help my cause. I became bitterly disappointed about the entire thing. I did not even open the *Bible*. It sat on my nightstand for quite a while. I would only move it when I was cleaning up my room.

The weeks went by. I was busy working and spending my spare time looking at food stores and trying to learn more about the poster I had seen at the doctor's office. I must have driven half way around the metropolitan area looking for a solution to my problem. What I discovered was that the store managers were not equipped with information on the produce in their stores and or how to prepare them. They did know that if you held certain foods in your hands without gloves they would spoil.

Now, the major cause of death is the food we eat; food plays a major part in life. I will say more about this later on.

I had not seen John and Mike for quite a while although I knew where to find John. Anytime I was able to touch base with them and tell them of my war stories and some of the ups and downs with the ladies.

They would say, "Zeke, you need to take a vacation on one of the islands and chill out with a few piña coladas for a couple of weeks and all your worries will disappear. And when you return you will be a new man."

We would then have a few drinks over it and have a good laugh.

By now I thought I had gathered enough information on fruits and vegetables, but I did not have the comfort of a kitchen where I lived. I had access to the kitchen downstairs but I did not want to inconvenience the landlord because it could have been a very messy project. I sought permission from Re, my girlfriend, to store some stuff in her refrigerator and she agreed, but her refrigerator could only hold so much. I pondered on that for a while.

Sometimes I would go across the street from where I lived to a friendly ice cream store where breakfast was prepared daily. I would go there and get some fresh-squeezed juice in the mornings; then for lunch I would have a slice of white bread and iceberg lettuce and at dinner I would have baked macaroni or some cooked greens. On days when I did not feel like eating food I would have bananas or grapes if they were in season. I thought I had it down perfectly.

I continued to work harder at the shop.

The guys would ask, "Zeke, why are you working so hard? Everyone is always on breaks and you keep pushing yourself."

The boss would come to the shop and asked, "Will this job be finished today?"

And I answered, "Yes."

He loved to hear that. He would send someone to the deli. "Go see if Zeke needs anything from the deli."

I would say, "Get me an ice tea or coke."

One Friday I got off from work—I was very tired—and I stopped off at Re. The kids were home from school and they were happy to see me. I had not been spending a lot of time with them and they were busy with their friends. Every Friday I used to take them to White Castle and then take them back to the house. They had this marvelous cat called Tinkle Bell; I did not like cats but this one used to snuggle up to me.

By the time Re got home the kids said, "Guess who is here?"

The mother said, "Who Sandy? He is back there?"

I came out and said, "Hello."

And she said, "What brings you here this time of the evening?"

In response, I said I dropped by to say hello. She told me I didn't look good and I told here I was tired and that it had been a rather long week for me. I asked whether I could stay the night.

Her response was, "I thought you were spending all your time with your other woman."

She finally said she had to think about it. I stayed for a while then I said goodnight to the kids. As I was about to leave she eventually relented and said I could spend the night. This was one night I did not want to be alone for some reason.

The following Sunday while catching up on the news, I came upon a large article on properties and top scale homes built to suit. I pondered on this article; things were going through my mind. I asked some of the guys if they knew anything about it but no one seemed to know anything about the sale of property in the Suffolk area. One Sunday I took a ride to the address given in the newspaper; clear instructions and directions were given on how to get there and the place was very easy to find. I did not know that Suffolk County had extended that far out. There were a lot of woods and forest areas. I thought Wyandanch was the extent of Suffolk County. We used to call it the boondocks; we used to say there was nothing out there and sometimes when you wanted to get rid of trash you drove out there and dumped it, so this was a new experience for me.

It was a beautiful day to go driving in the countryside. I finally got to the site; I noticed that I could smell fresh air and pine. I pulled into a parking lot where there were many people; there were also these beautiful model houses in the parking area. When you got out your car you merely walked into any one of the houses and took a tour. Someone was there to answer your questions so I looked around the different model homes for probably an hour or so.

I did not want to remain there too late just in case I could not find my way home. There were people from as far as Brooklyn and Queens who were seeking to move out to the countryside for a better life with their families. I overheard some of the conversations that were going on. The developers drove you to the locations where the properties were for sale. When it was my turn I was directed to see a gentleman in a particular room.

I walked into the room and there was a man in his seventies. He was very polite. He inquired what he could do for me and I informed him that I had seen the advertisement in the newspaper and I was seeking any further information on it. He explained that the homes were for young couples who wanted to start a family in a new community; and that the Government would provide assistance to obtain a home at low cost if I met the minimum requirement. I let him know that I didn't have a family; I was single. He was surprised because I was a Cushite and they had not seen Cushites here to purchase homes or properties; it was mostly Anglo-Saxons.

I inquired about the prices of the homes.

He said to me, "In speaking with you for the past few minutes you have been here, I can tell that you are a fine young man." Then he asked, "Do you have two thousand dollars?"

I sought to find out the purpose of the question and he indicated that because I was still a very young man, I could purchase land as an investment and build a house on it. He further advised that I could rent it out and move into it later on when I was ready to have a family. He mentioned that he had not seen a young man who had the ambition that I exhibited. I was anxious to know what I had to do next and he guided me every step of the way.

I was shown a piece of property. While we were on our way, the driver said to me, "The old man must really like you because this is a prime location and when it is built up it would be a little paradise."

From the time I got out of the car and we walked a little distance, he pointed out the piece of property to me. I fell in love with it right away. I walked a little way into the woods, taking deep breaths of the fresh air. He said that the bay was right down there, pointing to the area. There was one house next door and across the street there were six families; they were all black families on that block and they were there for some thirty years.

The gentleman eventually took me back to the office because he had to take other people to different locations to show them the various lots. When we arrived at the office the elderly gentleman was waiting for us and he inquired whether I liked the area and I said it was very nice. He reminded me that I was in a choice spot near everything and that the area was expanding. He assured me that he would not steer me in the wrong direction. He had all the papers already filled out. I did not have all the money on me so he promised to keep the paperwork on his desk until the following week. I told him if anything went wrong he wouldn't see me and I would call him and make other arrangements. We shook hands and I left.

On my way home, I thought about everything that transpired on that visit. I wondered whether I had made the right decision. I worried about if something went wrong after I handed over my two thousand dollars to the gentleman; I would be broke, I would not have a proper burial as I thought I should. I do not have to tell you that I could not sleep that night. I felt that I couldn't change my mind since I had given my word to this elderly man and shook his hand. It was my view that it was an honor to give someone your word and to keep your promise. You will be respected as a man your word was your honor.

I kept this deal a secret; I did not tell anyone, not even Re. I called the bank that Monday. I gave them my account number; the funds had even collected interest for the time it was there. I went back to work. The following Saturday I went to the bank and obtained a bank check. I felt that if anything went wrong, I could stop the check on Sunday. I left my room about noon and returned to the property developers to take care of business. When I got there I asked the gentleman if he remembered me.

He said, "Of course, I know you are a young man of your word. Some people don't return; you are a hard-working man. You have saved your money for something good; this is a sound investment, you can't go wrong."

I signed all the papers he put before me after he had explained everything. I handed over the check and he gave me his number. When I left that office I was twenty-seven thousand, five hundred dollars in debt and I did not know how I would repay it. The one good thing I thought about was that if I died, I didn't have to worry about repaying that money. I did not look at the Sunday newspaper for a while because I did not want to get in any further trouble.

By this time Re and myself were battling with our relationship. It was affecting me in a negative way. I thought several times about ending the relationship and move on but since she was always there when my health crisis occurred, I decided to try a little harder.

I eventually decided to take my friends' advice so I planned a vacation for the early part of 1977. The foundation work on the house was to begin in January of 1977 and I had wanted to be there when it started. We picked out an island that Re wanted to visit; it was the Paradise Island in the Bahamas.

We stayed on Paradise Island away from all the heavy traffic and the interaction with the everyday worries. The visit was twofold. Firstly, I was there hoping that my problems would disappear and secondly, to try to improve our relationship. We spent ten days in the Bahamas. We rented a small car to get around the island. Re wanted to visit all the gift and handicraft shops. We found out that Sidney Poitier was living on the island. He, however, did not go under his name. We found out where he lived and made an uninvited visit. It was a beautiful area with equally beautiful homes. There were these lovely palm trees on the property. It was a luxurious home, far in so that it was difficult to see the house from the roadway. He was not at home on that day. We were told that he was away on business but we were able to see the neighborhood. You had to be doing well financially to live there.

During the time of our visit to the Bahamas, Howard Hughes' yacht was also spending the winter months there—he had died the year before though—and I went down to the pier to get some pictures of the boat. I told the crew that I wanted to have a picture of Mr. Hughes' boat but I was not allowed to take pictures of the crew.

I knew that sea water was good for the body so while I was in the Bahamas I took advantage of taking long swims every morning to help strengthen my body, since it was a warm climate. I took advantage of all the tropical fruits that were available at that time. In the morning I would have freshly squeezed orange juice, not juice from a carton as we get here. I also had fruits like papaya, mango and soursop. For dinner I would have plantain, breadfruit, sweet potato (same as yam in the U.S.), yam and coconut water fresh from the tree (this is the liquid found in young green coconuts). When I went to the market, it was unbelievable to see the abundance of food that was not refrigerated.

Saturday we drove to the countryside enjoying the fresh air and the scenery and on our way back I heard the beat of drums in the distance.

At first I thought it was my imagination but once in a while the sounds will drift in our direction. Re was speaking to me but I was like curious as to where these sounds were coming from. As we got closer it was what I thought it was; it was the same kind of drum beat I had heard when I was a child; it does something to your soul.

The sound of this drum was getting louder and louder but I could not tell from where it was coming. However, as we got to a particular spot I stopped the car and we got out; I wanted to find out where the sound was coming from. Re thought it was something evil and I told her it was not.

She asked, "What do you know about Africa and voodoo?"

I laughed, because she did not know what she was speaking about.

We were on top of the roadway and I looked down this hill and there it was.

Let me explain a little here. Some of the roads were high above sea level and there were houses built in some of those dangerous areas below the roads. There were no railings so a driver who did not know the roads well could go over the hill on top of the houses thereby causing major damage and even death.

We looked down on this very small house and there were many people gathered. It seemed like friends and family. Someone observed us and signaled us to come on down. They showed us how to get to the bottom of the road by walking around. In other words, we had to leave the car on the roadway and walk alongside the road until we got to the lower part of the road before we got to the driveway.

It was a wedding ceremony. There were people dancing barefooted, including the bride and groom. It was a small house on stilts; there were people in the house and a tent was set up in the yard. It was not the tent you are accustomed seeing here at weddings. This tent was made of six or eight posts in the ground and covered with some branches. By the time we got there and were greeted, we told them that we were from the United States, but they already knew that we were tourists.

This was a rather unique experience. They were eating from the leaves of the banana plant with their bare hands. This may seem strange to some of us but it is their custom. They handed us the leaves with the food on it, which consisted of goat meat, rice, yam, green banana and plantain. Since I didn't eat meat, I ate everything else. Re was making faces at the food. The green plantain was cooked and pounded in a mortar and then rolled into a ball and then it was cut and served. One of the men asked Re to dance with him; although she struggled to keep up with their folk dance she thoroughly enjoyed it. A very delicious drink called sorrel was also served. It was very strong and you could have tasted the spices in it. As I said before, this was a very interesting experience.

After we were finished eating we got a chance to speak to the bride and groom. We did not know whether there was a church service or whether that part of the ceremony was performed at the house. I did not see anyone with a collar as that worn by a priest. The couple could have been in their forties, the bride was very attractive.

Throughout the entire time the elderly and all the other guests there were not fussing over anything. Everything was running smoothly. About half hour later we were getting ready to leave. It was a long day for us and it was quite humid. I had another cup of the sorrel drink then someone handed each of us another leaf, but this time it was wrapped and tied with string. We looked around and everyone was eating whatever it was. We untied the string and opened the banana leaf; there was a piece of yellow cake the size of a brownie. When I asked what it was I was told that it was corn pone. It was a very tasty and sweet delicacy. It was made by grating or grinding the dried corn to a course powder and then sugar, spices and other ingredients were added to it. It was placed on the leaf, which was then folded, tied and placed in boiling water to cook for a while. They called it "Payme." It is one of the staple foods on the island.

That evening after we returned to the hotel I thought we would stay in that night and relax but Re said she was on vacation and she wanted to go out. We got dressed and went to the casino; it was very crowded. Now, I was not a gambling man, especially in casinos but I purchased fifty dollars worth of chips. I played a few and had no luck and so I decided that they already had too much of my money and I was not going to spend anymore. Re was so excited playing all the various machines so I did not interrupt her fun.

About one o'clock in the morning I told her it was time for us to go but she insisted that she wouldn't leave until she got back her money, so I left her at the casino and went back to the hotel. Later that morning, I went to get some breakfast and she offered to pay despite my insistence that I would pay. We both knew that things were not working out as we hoped. We eventually ended our trip and returned home.

I wanted to visit the construction site to see how far the work had progressed. However, soon after I returned from the vacation I fell ill and was laid up at Denise's house trying to recover. Everyone was looking for me. It seemed as though everyone in the town of Brookhaven was searching for me.

The job wanted to know why I was not reporting to work. When I recuperated two weeks later, I went to my residence; the landlord wanted to know if I was in the hospital again. I told him I was sick and at a friend's house. He handed me a phone number to call. I also had to go to the post office to sign for some certified letters. When I opened the letters, one of them informed me that the house was finished and they needed my signature on some checks. The company that built the house could not get paid until I signed those documents. The next set of mail informed me that the house had burnt down. It seemed as though I was going through one problem after another and I did not know how to solve them. Also, there were a few suits against me by the town of Brookhaven for debris that was spread along the county road and I had to pay the county for cleaning up the mess.

I called the number that my landlord had given me and a young lady answered. I said to her, "My name is Mr. Sandy; I understand you all were looking for me."

She said, "Mr. Sandy please stay on the line, don't go."

Eventually a gentleman came on the line and asked me if I could come out there today and I told him I could not. They tried to explain what they think happened with the house. I told them I had been going through a lot over the past few weeks but I promised I would be there the following day. That night I did not sleep. The next day I prepared myself for the worst. I wondered what else could go wrong: Re and I had broken up by this time; Denise was pregnant; my house had burnt down before I could set foot inside and the town had filed a lawsuit against me.

When I got to the office there was coffee, donuts and bagels laid out. The officials were happy to see me because the checks had to be signed by me so that the contractors and everyone else including the attorney could be paid. The attorney said they would handle the lawsuit and other legal matters. I also had insurance on the property.

I signed all the paperwork they put in front of me then they informed me that they would move me from that spot. That was a shocker to me because I really loved that location. I questioned why I had to move but they did not give me a good enough reason. Instead, they promised to give me more property wherever I chose. They drove me around for about half a day showing me many choice parcels of land but everywhere they took me, I did not like. They finally brought me back to the office and tried to convince me that the locations were all the same but I was not swayed. You see, I had fallen in love with the first location. Before I left they asked whether I would change my mind and I said no.

Now why do I mention these things to you? When you are suffering with any kind of illness, you need to be free from all stress-related problems because stress could lead to death. Here I was, a man who had endured many years of health problems and yet I had to take on a new kind of experience, which I did not have the strength or the energy to fight. This new kind of disease, I call them disease because they bring no joy, love or happiness in your life, but if you could survive these onslaughts they can strengthen you.

By the way, when you are experiencing problems, running away or taking a vacation does not make things better or change things around. Wherever you go your worries go with you; they never leave your mind; you think about them, especially at nights. The best way to deal with your situation is to face it head on.

There I was, all broken up over all my issues and the attorneys said, "I will take care of it."

I found myself in another predicament when Denise announced that she was pregnant. I kept to my room; I did not want to go over to her house anymore, but the damage was already done. I worried about passing on my illness to the baby. I did not want the baby to undergo the same problems I was experiencing. When I thought about all those babies I saw at the clinic and what they were going through, I could not bear for that child to go through that ordeal for the rest of his days. I thought about her having an abortion, but I knew that she would not agree to that because she was strong in her faith and the Catholic priest would not allow such a thing. All sorts of things came into my mind but I finally decided that whatever happened I would have to face it.

I questioned what kind of life I could give that child. After all, I was a man who could barely take care of himself; I lived partially on the system and could only work when I was able to. I did not think I was ready for this kind of new experience and responsibility, but I knew whatever it was I had to face it. I kept hoping that the baby would not have the same sickle cell trait or the sickle cell disease. I kept working to put some extra money aside for when the baby came. I had a breather because the house was not ready for me to move into after it was burnt down so I had some time to make some extra money. My biggest fear at that time was that I would fall sick once again.

I found a shop on the North Shore where I did some repair work at night. I took the job; they knew me and the owner was impressed with my work. However, it turned out that I found it difficult to work there because the owner had five sons who fought constantly; it was frustrating at times but I needed the extra cash. I would finish late at night and then had to get up early for my day job. Sometimes I would be tired but I would strive to keep up.

Although I tried to eat a balanced diet of lean foods, fruits and vegetables, I was setting up myself for a big fall. Everything looked good during the few months of working two jobs. I felt proud of myself because I was making the extra cash I wanted. I slept all day on Sundays. On my day job, I worked extra time to get the work out on time. I was going along drinking water and lemonade. By this time I had stopped drinking soft drinks.

One night, I stopped by Re to see how the kids were doing because I did not see them for quite a while. I took them some of their favorite food: burgers and fries. They wanted to know whether I was sick again and I explained that I was just working a lot more hours. They stated that I looked terrible. Re did not know that Denise was pregnant with my child, but I did not think it was a good time to break that news to her. I, however, mentioned to her that I was in the process of buying my own home so I was working more hours to make the extra money. She questioned whether I was buying a house for my other woman, because I was not in any good health to own a home.

I did not put up an argument with her because it would only lead to the same thing as always, fighting. The kids, however, wanted to know if they could come live with me.

I said, "Anytime."

Well, it wasn't long before the proverbial lightening struck. I became ill once again. This time, the headache was so severe I felt as though my temple would explode. I wrapped a wet towel around my head. I was extremely terrified because I thought my time had finally come.

Do you remember the free *Bible* I received through the mail when I ordered the three medical books for one dollar? Well, I placed it between my legs and squeezed. I prayed, as I never did before.

I wanted to make things right with everyone who I thought I had done wrong and to ask for forgiveness. I really thought that night was my last. I thought about the baby on the way; I thought about the unfinished house; I thought about the promise I made at the hospital. Everything was slowly disappearing in front of me.

That night I would bite down on my pillow to keep from screaming out and waking the roommate on the other side and the landlord downstairs. I rolled, kicked and dripped from sweat, holding on to dear life. I took a few of the Advil; I did not want to take too much of the medication. My mouth was very dry and had a bitter taste. I kept swallowing my saliva so as to wet my throat. I went through this agony during the night just hoping to see the dawn of a new day, which I was not sure I was going to accomplish. I thought about going to the hospital that night, but I felt that I would rather die at home.

I no longer had the burial money because it went into the down payment for the house. Also, I could not endure lying in the hospital bed listening to those squeaky wagons all through the night taking the dead to the morgue. I therefore decided to take the painkillers and go through the suffering.

Have you ever been confined to the hospital and you could only lie on one side at a time because of the number of injection sites on your rear and when there was no other place they started on the thighs and your sides? No? Well, that was a very painful situation and I had been through all this on many occasions so I decided to persevere.

As you can tell, I made it through the night. There was a calmness that I felt in the morning. I took the *Bible* and I started to read from the beginning. It said that "God created man in his own image," and "God formed man of the dust of the ground, and breathed into his nostrils the breath of life; and man became a living soul." And "eastward in Eden" the Great I Am planted a garden and gave it to Adam to "dress it" and to keep it and the trees bearing food and seeds for food and medicine.

It dawned on me then that this was what I must do. I flipped through some of the other pages and I saw where the children of Israel were complaining about the food they were not getting anymore like the melons, leeks, garlic and cucumbers. It seemed as though a door opened in my brain.

I remembered all the things my grandfather and my father, Altino Jeremiah, had taught me about food. Everything then began to fall into place. Then I remembered the picture I had seen at the doctor's office. I realized that I had been taught well about the land and food, but somehow I neglected these things. I questioned why I did not remember such valuable information about food that I was exposed to as a child. I was puzzled and I became confused. This did not make sense. I know I was not dreaming because I was wide awake. Yes, my mind was not all there but I was conscious enough to know what was taking place.

I wondered why these foods were not used for medicinal purposes. Why were these foods not used for healing the human body instead of drugs, injections and all kinds of potions? This was information that the Great I Am, The Great Creator of the universe who created all things gave Moses to record.

I also read in another chapter where John said that the herb would be used to heal the nation. He also said that the same food was also for meat. I stopped reading and closed the Bible. I mentioned earlier that I used to stake out some of the grocery stores in the wee hours of the morning in order to find out all I needed to know about the different kinds of foods and where they came from. However, it dawned on me that I was going about it the wrong way. I had to go back to the beginning where I was taught about all the land, soil, water, right food, wrong food, what to eat and what not to eat.

Everything was coming back to me like if it were yesterday. I became very excited about my newfound knowledge. I was not fully recovered because I was still very weak. I had to hold on to anything in order to get to the bathroom. This disease weakened me considerably whenever it came over me; it was a very terrifying feeling.

ATTEMPTING TO FEED MYSELF

At last I received a letter informing me that the house was finished; it took about four months to complete. I was advised by the developers they would not be responsible for any theft on the property after they had finished so I had to move in as soon as possible. The process of moving was very tiresome despite the fact that I did not have many personal belongings to take to the new house.

The landlord allowed me to leave some of my stuff until I was able to pick them up. It was also a way for me to stop by and see him when I was in the area. I finally got the keys and moved into an unfurnished house. There were no curtains for the windows and no bed and other furniture. I used my shirts as shades for the windows at night to keep the moonlight from my face and sheets were spread on the bare floor where I slept. But guess what? I finally had my own kitchen. I was ready to take on the task of preparing my own meals. I was now ready as I would ever be.

From a child I had known about water and the proper water to drink. Speaking about water, my house was one of the first to have pipe-borne water in the area. Previously, everyone in the neighborhood used water from wells until later on when water lines were run through the side street and connected from the main line from my driveway. I have not drunk tap water for thirty-one years; that is since the house was built in 1977. I only use that water for washing, bathing and cleaning. The only types of water I drink are pure spring water and distilled water.

One week when I knew the semi-fresh fruits and vegetables were available, I went out and bought some. I placed one cap of bleach in a sink of lukewarm water and washed the fruits and vegetables thoroughly. I dried them and place them in bags. After three days, what I had not used I would dispose of them. I needed fruits and vegetables that were as fresh as possible. Any food that has been in the refrigerator for more than three days is not good for the system.

I would drive far and wide to get the best stocks that I needed. I learned many years ago that the local stores would carry everything that you possible needed but not quality stuff. There were no books on sickle cell that I knew of which provided knowledge on how to heal the body. The information was locked up in my head and it did not surface until it was revealed to me after reading certain passages in the *Bible*.

In the mornings, I would eat whatever fruits were in season. In the case of watermelons, I would eat the meat and drink the juice in abundance. I needed to use organic juices to bathe the cells. I ate cloves of garlic with my meals. I ate garlic until you could smell it on me.

My clothing used to smell of garlic and then I knew it was working. The garlic was used to open the pores of the skin so that the toxic waste could come out from the body and also help to build up my resistance. I cut up the vegetables in small pieces so that they would be easily masticated and digested. I ate the raw vegetables until my mouth got sore from chewing some of the hard stuff-carrots, cabbage some of the leafy hard vegetables—but the garlic would heal my mouth overnight. Then I would drink "bush" teas; this is where the leaves of certain plants are steeped in hot water for a while before drinking the liquid. Around this time herbal tea bags were not in abundance.

I experienced my parents and grandparents drinking bush teas made from peppermint leaves, sage leaves, bay leaves, comfrey leaves, Eden Green tea. I usually drank these teas very strong sweetened with a little honey, the raw kind, or wild. I would also get the honeycomb, remove the bees and eat the honey in the morning. I also took the aloe plant, scraped out the gel and added it to juices. This resulted in frequent bowel movements and also was beneficial to my digestive system. In the morning I would take the juice of two lemons in hot water to wash out my liver and kidneys.

There were many other products that I needed but I did not know where to locate them. I needed a certain kind of butter made from the milk of goats. I did not find any right away. However, I found someone who raised goats and sold the young kids for the holy days. I met with him and he promised to give me when the goats were breastfeeding in the spring. It was a happy moment for me to locate someone at last who could assist in this area.

Apart from human milk, the goats' milk is the only milk that is good for the human digestive system. Goats' milk, without treating it, has the right kind of butter for the stomach lining and the lubricant for the stomach walls. It is also the best known for the amount of enzymes that are very beneficial for the digestive system and small intestines and also provide many other nutrients for the body.

I continued to work diligently looking for ways to make my task easier. I had two hills to climb: one, how to get rid of the wax on the foods and two, a better way to obtain quality foods. In my county, there were many farms that grew corn, potatoes, cabbage, watermelons, tomatoes and other vegetables and fruits. On these farms some type of fertilization was used on the soil for faster growth as well as to enhance the soil. They sold these produce to some of the grocery stores where I purchased my produce. This was an uphill battle for me because if I didn't get the right foods my efforts would have been in vain.

I, therefore, continued to search around for more natural foods and I found out that there were a few health-food stores that carried some organic vegetables. I was instructed to look in my local telephone yellow pages. I didn't know that I had one in the village where I lived so I was thrilled when I found one. It was not too far from my home so I visited and asked many questions. The owner was not too co-operative; she did not seem thrilled to have a new customer. First, I thought it was just me. I did not want to do business with her but the store was close to my residence and it had some of the things I needed. Sometimes I would travel far to get my vegetables because I was determined to accomplish the goal of reclaiming my life.

In the meanwhile, I would visit Denise and sometimes I spent the night at her place. At this time her stomach was like a medium-sized watermelon. One day she visited me at work and on her way home, she was involved in an accident—apparently she stopped at a stop sign and a motorcar hit her from behind. She telephoned me later to let me know what had happened; I was thankful that both she and the baby she was carrying were okay.

My greatest mission was to keep on searching for quality green vegetables because the juices from these vegetables are required to travel down through the bile duct to the cells to feed them with the proper nutrients. It was an uphill fight in those days to find quality food. Through my search, I found out that these food stores did not know much about quality foods. Some people with whom I spoke never ate vegetables but they would consume a lot of meat, bread, pasta, fried foods, cola drinks, ice cream and lots of other junk food and they honestly believed that they were eating healthy. I went further east and there were more problems in that area; they had many wine tasting events on Sundays. Tents would be set up and customers would travel over a hundred miles to sample the wines to determine who had the better quality. There were other farmers growing vegetables such as corn, potatoes, peppers, greens, beetroot and lettuce among others.

There was no break for me in sight but I continued to preserve because I knew sooner or later there would be a breakthrough. Time was of the essence for me because, according to the doctors, I did not have much of it left and the baby would be born soon. We already had names picked out for him because we knew it was going to be a boy, although everyone else thought that it was going to be a girl. My only hope was that it would be a healthy baby.

I noticed that after a few months I was not as tired as I used to be. I thought that I was just having a few good days. Although I wanted to jump for joy over this little bit of success, I tried to keep calm. I also noticed that the rashes and dry skin were disappearing. I noticed that I had more endurance in whatever I did so I persevered relentlessly with the regime I had started.

I was now searching for a way to separate the juice from the pulp and the vegetables. I tried pounding the vegetables in a rag, but I was making a mess. I remember seeing mortars when I visited the islands. These are bowl-shaped vessels hollowed out from tree stumps in which substances are crushed with a pestle. They come

Ezekiel Sandy

in varying sizes. It stood about three feet high. The pestle is also made from wood; it looks like a baseball bat but much heavier. Whatever is to be crushed is put in the mortar and pounded with the pestle. I searched the county but no one knew what I was speaking about. Today, however, they can be found in some health food stores. These are little bowls used to grind herbs and spices. Although it was a challenge to locate the right tools to crush the foods for easier absorption, I was determined to overcome all the obstacles that were in my way.

I increased my daily allowance of vegetables. I also increased my garlic intake until the odor was coming through my skin. I needed to sweat out much of the poisons from my liver so that my kidney could help expel some of the poisons. I drank the herbal teas that I knew were beneficial to me. I was forced to use the dry leaves because I could not get the fresh leaves.

Herbal teas are valuable for cleansing the body and strengthening the organs. I also scraped the gel from the aloe vera plant and blended it with juice and drank it. Now let me tell you, this does not have a pleasant taste. I would hold my nose and swallow it. I used the aloe plant for the hard working digestive system, to assist in the healing of the sore tract and to help clean the small intestines from the buildup of debris.

It was almost time for my check-up at the clinic; I did not know what to expect. I did not want to display any signs that I was doing anything outside of what the doctors prescribed

---

Ezekiel Sandy

in varying sizes. It stood about three feet high. The pestle is also made from wood; it looks like a baseball bat but much heavier. Whatever is to be crushed is put in the mortar and pounded with the pestle. I searched the county but no one knew what I was speaking about. Today, however, they can be found in some health food stores. These are little bowls used to grind herbs and spices. Although it was a challenge to locate the right tools to crush the foods for easier absorption, I was determined to overcome all the obstacles that were in my way.

I increased my daily allowance of vegetables. I also increased my garlic intake until the odor was coming through my skin. I needed to sweat out much of the poisons from my liver so that my kidney could help expel some of the poisons. I drank the herbal teas that I knew were beneficial to me. I was forced to use the dry leaves because I could not get the fresh leaves.

Herbal teas are valuable for cleansing the body and strengthening the organs. I also scraped the gel from the aloe vera plant and blended it with juice and drank it. Now let me tell you, this does not have a pleasant taste. I would hold my nose and swallow it. I used the aloe plant for the hard working digestive system, to assist in the healing of the sore tract and to help clean the small intestines from the buildup of debris.

It was almost time for my check-up at the clinic; I did not know what to expect. I did not want to display any signs that I was doing anything outside of what the doctors prescribed

106

because this would upset them. When I got to the clinic that day and I looked at all the kids, especially those with the sickle cell disease, I felt hurt because I knew what they were going through. Some of them were crying because they couldn't bear the pain and their parents looked so helpless. It was not a pleasant sight to behold. I cannot say whether any of these children are alive today.

When my name was called and I went into the office to see my doctor, she looked at me as though something was wrong. Yes, something was wrong because I did not look the same; I looked better than the last time she saw me. She was excited so she called another doctor to take a look at me, then they conversed in another office. They had seen some improvement in me; not much, but enough to raise their eyebrows.

She was happily told me, "You are doing well with the medication."

I said, "Yes, it is working."

I did not mention anything that I was doing. I did not want to alarm them. One thing I learned from my past experience with taking medication and engaging in alternative treatments was not to alarm the doctors by letting them know that you were doing anything other than what they told you to do. I learned to keep my mouth shut and didn't let the doctor know that I was not following her advice.

I remember once a doctor instructed me to take a particular medication at a certain times of the day, more than twice per day. However, the first time I took the medicine I became very ill and vomited. I stopped taking the medication there and then. When I went back to him he asked me whether I was taking the medicine and I answered truthfully that I did not take them. He was not even interested in an explanation; he became very angry with me and I noticed changes in our relationship. At times when I went to see him I felt that he did not want to see me, so I learned from that experience. Whatever I was doing on my own to improve my health, I kept it to myself.

So when I went to the clinic and the doctor saw the improvement, I was given higher doses of medication. I must tell you that as I cleared the hospital area, I would open the car window and throw them out. If I was given an injection in the buttocks I would wait until it wore off and I would go right back and continue the regimen of drinking herbal teas to rid my system of the drugs.

This was a time for me to rejoice. Many good things were happening. On October 12, 1977 a son was born to Denise and Zeke; he was born in the Nassau County Medical Center, the same hospital where I was hospitalized with my health ordeal. When I first laid eyes on him it was a joyful occasion for me and I knew that I had to overcome all the odds. My greatest fear was that he might have the disease. God knows I did not want him to go through the same suffering that I was experiencing. It was too early to tell but there were other problems that the doctors were concerned about, which I would not go into now.

There was one thing I did not have and that was time. Was I ready to die at this time? No. What story would he be told about me? Would he learn about his father from some half truths and by pictures? No, I wanted more; I wanted to hold him and do things with him. Those were questions I kept asking myself so I knew that I had to overcome this challenge; I had something to live for. When looking at this baby I could see the joy in his face. I now had an extra drive. I would travel far and wide looking for information on sickle cell. There was no information on curing the disease, only medication to manage the pain. I realized that I was on the right road by adopting this new and healthy lifestyle that was required to overcome the challenge I was undergoing.

I kept pushing myself because my parents always told us, "Hard work does not kill, it makes you stronger." I spent my spare time searching for books that had information on diseases because I knew I would not find the answer in the medical field. I read information about diseases such as chicken pox, measles, malaria typhoid and lumbago and they all followed practically the same pattern. One of the things I learned was that life is in the blood; that what causes the destruction in the blood has to come from something we ingest in some form into the body because the Creator said that His creation was perfect and good.

If the blood is not clean and a mosquito bites you or you drink dirty water, then you could contract malaria. If a tick bit you and the blood is not clean that poison will get into the blood and affect the central nervous system and cause a chronic imbalance in your body.

MOTIVATION IN TIME OF SICKNESS

When I learned those lessons I started to apply those principles by finding ways to clean the blood. It took me some time to discover these answers and then how to correct the situation. It was not an easy task. As my understanding grew, I began to see things much clearer. Sometimes my heart would race and I took deep breaths to calm myself. I kept on eating green vegetation and struggled to find a way to extract the liquids from these foods; I did not give up. Yes, some days I got frustrated with myself and I would go without food for a day or so, punishing myself, then I would slowly pull myself back on track and kept fighting off all the evil or negative thoughts that sought to overwhelm me.

One of the most destructive things is our thoughts and mind. The reason I could relate to this is because, as I stated before, I tried to commit suicide. I learned a great deal about coping with life in dealing with this disease. I also learned never to give up even when things looked bleak.

When I was at Mercy Hospital I used to observe the painful expression on my friend's face; he would clutch his weak hands and he would say, "I am going to make it." He was determined to recover, but unfortunately he did not; he had hope and that was most important.

The other thing I learned with illness is that you need motivation; you need something to take your mind off the pain; you need something to boost your self-esteem; you need something to quicken your thoughts; something to preserve your mind—the ocean, the ripple of the waves crashing down on the rocks. When I think about the energy that is produced from water, it gives me goose bumps. When I think back, way back about thirty years ago when I used to go diving in the coral waters in St. John's, Virgin Islands, there were those pretty colored fish we called Butter Fish. You should see how these fish just got a burst of new energy to escape from the larger fish that wished to make them a meal. You had to really be there to experience the energy these Butter Fish had. Water brings you new life. I would reflect on those good times when I needed that bit of spark.

My mother told a story to the older ones once, about my father who at one time was a fisherman. Apparently, he used to take the bread that she made, out to sea and feed the dolphins and when he returned, he used to relate the joy he got from watching these dolphins perform in the ocean. Sometimes those waves would rise six to twelve feet high and these mammals would shoot over this small boat and plunge back into the waters. They were so energetic that sometimes he felt like jumping in.

New birth could also motivate you. I remember when my son was born just to see that little baby with such an innocent look on his face as though he was asking, "Where am I? I am not used to this; everything seems strange."

When I looked at him it put a spark in me that made me want to live at all costs. I did not want anything to get in my way to prevent me from overcoming the odds.

Nineteen hundred and seventy-seven was a very interesting year; there were many ups and downs and a lot of overcoming. There was an abundance of joy in surmounting all the challenges and entering this new year of 1978. I was very upbeat, looking forward to all good things and being involved with the three boys: David, Dexter and Darrell. They also provided a spark in my life. Dexter would spend the weekends and also some of the weekdays with me. I would take him to school and then pick up him and the rest of his brothers and drop by to say hello to Re.

I never forgot that Re was there for me during my ordeal in fighting off this disease. As a young lad I was taught to never forget people who helped you when you were in need and it was not fair to her and especially the kids. It seemed as though she wanted to give the relationship another try and she spoke to me about it. I gave it some thought but I just could not walk away from the new baby. I remember one day she went out and bought a toy and tried to persuade me to give it to the mother and tell her that the relationship was over, but I just could not bring myself to do that. It was another one of those points where when you think you are having a smooth ride everything just gets topsy-turvy again. I kept seeing that little face so full of joy. This went on for a few months but I had to let it go. My health was beginning to affect me slowly. I was becoming mentally weak. In such a short time many things were falling apart. I had to take things into my own hands quickly because I did not want to fall into a stupor. Based on that decision, I continued to thrive.

I spent the year of 1978 experimenting with different kinds of treatments. One such treatment involved the use of the aloe vera plant I would purchase from the garden stores. I would take them home and split the plant down the center and I scooped out as much of the gel as I could into a bowl and cut up the flesh into small pieces. I would drink about a half cup of this slimy, bitter stuff. Boy, this tasted like hell! I followed this up with either some apple juice or orange juice but the taste of aloe would be in my mouth for a few days.

Well, you may ask, why did I do that? It was because my system had been so weakened from this disease that I needed to put some of the spark back into the cells. I needed a greater intake of vitamins and minerals and to restore the nutrients in the digestive system.

As I said before, I drank a lot of herbal teas. I stayed away from black tea and coffee since these were high in stimulants and not beneficial to the liver. By taking so much medication it had affected my liver so I had to find herbal teas that would help detoxify the bad liver enzymes. I used teas such as Milk Thistle, Yellow Dock, Violet and Red Clover because they helped remove some of the harmful wastes that the liver tried to rid the body of.

Remember, these were just used for experimentation to see the effect they would have on my health. I tried different things such as drinking castor oil. I would just put the bottle to my mouth and swallow the stuff. All the things I remembered my parents giving us as medicine when we were children were motivation to me. I also tried fasting by going without food and water for three days, which is very effective in any health problem.

Over the course of a few months I took things into my own hands without informing anyone about what I was doing for fear that they would think I was endangering myself. For me, however, it was the will to live so that I could enjoy life for a longer period of time. That was my main goal, to keep fighting to stay alive.

I would eavesdrop at a few health food stores to see whether anyone had any information that would improve my health. It was the same old stories I was hearing, about these Chinese herbs that could cure all mankind's troubles. Then I heard about the herbs that the Native Americans used for years. So I decided to look into these bits of information but was unable to get anywhere with that, so I would take up the

Bible, my Comforter, and look to see what I had missed. After all, it was "The Comforter" that was restoring all my knowledge about the things that were missing in my health.

By reading the *Bible*, I found where "The Comforter" said that the herbs are for healing the nation.

I asked myself, "What herbs?" "What nation?"

This was a challenge because I did not know how to go about searching for these herbs. The only lead I got was back at the health-food store where bits and pieces of information were contained either in books or newsletters. So I had to continue to look to the Source because even if I had seen the herbs that were used when I was a child in my backyard, I would not have remembered or recognized them. Also, I could not approach my friends on this matter because they would have known that I was not on the medication, so I therefore had to continue to work alone and keep my actions to myself.

On the job, I would raise certain conversations on herbs with the South American brothers. They would talk about the cactus flower their parents used for healing. They talked about the bush teas that they drank and the papaya used for internal problems but there was no sound information on which I could rely.

From my experience, I know that you can gain knowledge from others if you listen very carefully to what has been said. You take the good stuff and leave the bad stuff. My goal was not only to beat this disease, but also be able to understand the nature of it and how I could help others to overcome it or even to manage the pain.

This disease brings a different kind of pain; it is a pain I never could get used to. I can't really explain it. The pain seemed to attack every nerve and organ in the body; I would feel so helpless and weak it would take, sometimes, a couple of weeks to recover. By being on so many medications, constipation was a problem. Sometimes it felt as though there was a plug driven in my rectum to stop anything from excreting. When I went to the bathroom to relieve myself, I would make all these facial expressions and my eyes would be tearing just to overcome the ordeal. Then I remembered that as a child when the grapefruit was in season, we used to squeeze the juice of several grapefruits in a large container, strained the seeds out and sweeten with brown large grained sugar or blackstrap molasses and that used to move our bowels. It is amazing how medication could close up the organs in the body and bind them like cement.

During this ordeal in my life there were some things to smile about like now the little fellow was running around like nothing was happening in his world. He continued to cause us to smile each day and this was one of the important strengths that brought me through this nightmare.

Betsy, my car, and I would travel on the weekend to different locations searching for answers. I heard about a botanical garden in the neighboring county so I decided to check to see if I could recognize any of the herbs there that I knew as a young lad. I took a trip to this botanical garden one day and when I arrived, there were many cars parked on the street. Many of the couples were holding hands and everyone was looking down like they lost something. As I got to the area, there were all these different kinds of plants and small trees on the ground; they all had nametags on them. There was also someone there to give you a bit of information about the flowers and the plants such as their origin. It looked more like a plantain field to me. I did not recognize many of the names of these plants but I was hoping to learn something new before the day was over.

I listened to information on the plants, for example, what location of the house the plants should be placed to get the best sunlight during the day. After hours of browsing in the field I stumbled on some herbs, the local species like rosemary and thyme. I realized that the thyme I knew, the leaves were broad, but the leaves on this plant were narrower. There were no herb books available to me at that time. I learned though that there was a lot of knowledge available about plants. Some of the persons there that day were very interested in the information they could acquire. There was a sense of love in the air; lots of smiles and head shaking and the beautiful layout of the garden with all the various kinds of plants. It was just amazing.

As I said a few times before, my journey in the search for answers to my issues continued. I went through some of the books at the local library to see if there was any new information but it was the same old story: just the same books on pain management, nothing on the cure for sickle cell disease or sickle cell trait. I maintained my daily regimen with the foods that would help to restore the organs, the tissues and the liver since they were under so much abuse from the medication and the devitalized foods that I had eaten earlier in my life.

FASTING

One day I received a letter—now I must tell you that I got very few of these. This was not an ordinary letter. It had about three stamps on it so I turned it over and realized that it was from the state of Wisconsin. Although I was a little afraid, I was anxious to open it; it was a letter from my Mom who I had not seen or heard from for over a decade.

Apparently, she was now living in Milwaukee. My heart leaped for joy. I could not read the letter immediately because I was too emotional. I took some time to calm myself. It was one of the best bits of news I had in a long time and it came at the right time, when I was down and out from the circle of iron to get good news from a mother. The other bit of good news, of course, was the birth of my son but this letter gave me new life. I thought about all those years we had not been in contact with each other. I found out that my mother thought that I was killed in the war in Vietnam but she never gave up looking for me, so for over thirty years I was supposed to be dead. Yes, I had been dead in the flesh with this horrible disease.

I finally read the letter over and over and tears flowed freely down my face. There was a lot more that was written in that letter that I do not wish to discuss at this time. I will touch on some of the highlights later in other chapters. This letter gave me the will and the extra energy to go on. It seemed as though every time I was about to fall, something or someone was there to catch me or to motivate me to keep me on going.

By this time, I had about one year and six months to live, according to the experts, and it did not matter how I tried not to think about it, it was always there in the back of my mind that my time was running out. This kept me on my toes to go out and search to discover that cure as quickly as I could.

There were times that I forgot how far I had gotten with the changing of my eating habits. Without making those changes, I would not have come this far, but my goal was to succeed so that I could help anyone who suffered from this disease. I saw the number of babies, young children and teenagers who were stricken with this ailment. Sometimes I wondered how many of them survived as long as I did and actually overcame this deadly killer. I saw enough to know that many of them did not make it, like the fifteen-year-old girl. There were times when I offered my help to her family, but since I was not a doctor they were not interested because they were under medical care. Unfortunately, this young girl died a few years later.

My health had improved tremendously so much so that at the clinic, the doctors were impressed with the medication because they thought it was effective. As a result, I was not required to attend the clinic once a week anymore, but every two weeks, and then subsequently, once a month unless there were complications or they wanted to try a new drug. Other than that, I was working my way out of the hospital and outpatient clinic.

One of the things I was looking at was fasting. I did not have full knowledge about fasting and I did not want to experiment with something I knew nothing about. I read about fasting in the *Bible*, which I referred to as "The Comforter," because that book gave me comfort in my loneliness and during those periods of great agony. Some of the most agonizing moments I suffered were when the pain hit me from all sides. I read and reread the verses until I understood them.

I used the sunset and the evening of one day and the morning of the following day as the first day. I ate my last meal before sunset and I would use that evening and the other morning as the first day. I would go for three days without food and water and on the evening of the fourth day, I would drink warm herbal teas and some light fruits such as grapes and watermelon because they are easier to digest. Also, I would not eat later than eight in the evening.

During those periods I was very weak, lightheaded and my stomach felt as though there was a deep hole in it. I also noticed that my bowel movement was different from that of regular bowel movements. I also felt a lot lighter. I knew that by fasting I was getting rid of lots of the toxins in my body that caused my problems through the years. I repeated this process after a few months. The most difficult time to fast was during the summer months because the days seemed longer and during those hot days I got very thirsty but I tried to conserve my energy. As I continued to fast, I became better at it.

One of my worst experiences while fasting was on a cold January day. There was a lot of snow that night and all through the night the plows were clearing the roads. I lived very close to the street and my driveway was blocked with a mound of snow I would have to clear before I could get to the street. It was a twenty-foot driveway. This task would take a lot of energy. I was in my third day of the fast; I started to work from in front of the doorway and by the time I reached the middle of the driveway I felt very dizzy, weak and I began to perspire profusely. I bent over the shovel and tried to compose myself; I was able to get back into the house and into bed because I was very nauseous. I eventually headed to the bathroom where I vomited only liquids. This went on for about half an hour. For the rest of that week I was very weak. I drank some of the herbal teas, took a tablespoon of raw unheated honey as well as ate bee pollen as part of my meal. It was a very terrifying feeling for me that day. For the rest of that week I consumed some broth to replace some of the minerals that I had lost during that episode. The broth consisted of carrot, celery, onions, parsley and garlic cloves.

The reason for me using this type of broth was that it had been known by my grandparents that when the body was injured, in order to help bring it back into balance then a liquid that has minerals: calcium, potassium, selenium, silicon, manganese and iron. This broth should be taken warm; neither hot nor cold. The cooking temperature should be no more than 1.30 degrees Fahrenheit.

As I went along this journey I gained more and more confidence in what I did because I built on what I learned from my experience, from parents and grandparents and, most of all, "The Comforter" helped me to be disciplined in what I did. I received no other help; as a matter of fact, no one knew what I was doing, because I confided in no one.

One of the things I experienced during my many stays at hospitals was the loneliness that comes with the illness and also being around negative people. My friend who was dying from cancer refused to listen to the other guy next to him with all his negative conversations.

He used to say to me, "Don't listen to him; he will make you more sick."

In his own way, that guy was trying to cheer us up but he did not know that it was damaging to the rest of the patients in that room. He was the only one on that ward who tried to cheer up the other patients by making negative remarks to everyone. So I learned to channel my thoughts in the right direction.

There was a small bay close to where I lived; it was a ten-minute walk from my house. I would go there to watch the seagulls dive into the water trying to catch herrings. I thought about how hard they had to work for their food. When they were full they would play with each other and after a while I would find myself smiling because these seagulls would land on the pier and start pecking at each other. Then I guess the male would chase away those that were creating problems, but at the end of the day they seemed like a happy family.

Let me jump ahead a few years for a second. In nineteen eighty-one I found out that some of my sisters were informed about my health through Re, my ex-girlfriend. Now, Re and I would talk now and again; my relationship with the boys was still intact. In fact, we always had a healthy relationship. We would do many things together. We went to the movies; when they had events at school I would be there. For instance, when David was in high school, he used to play the flute in the school band and when they had concerts I was cheering him on. Darrell was in Lacrosse and he was very good at it; his team won many of their games. Dexter, he was a bit different; he was more an outdoor type. He liked to play the field; he was a little on the wild side and although he wanted to go away to college in Texas, we supported him. So we were all a very close family, despite all my health problems and everything else.

In 1975, one winter morning I went in to work. Now, this is the same job I held with the same company since the spring of 1975, the Chevrolet dealer. The only difference was that I was not in the union. Since the company closed the body shop and leased it to a private individual, I was the only one who was kept on because of my experience, commitment to the company and the quality of my work. There was no heat in the body shop; the heating unit was in the large building but the ducts for the heating system were in different sections of the building. I was asked to fix the heater. Now, this building was very huge with a height of 20 to 30 feet. I had to use a ladder to reach the unit to determine whether it was a job I could handle.

Well, by the time I got to the top of the ladder and was checking out the thermostat to see if it was malfunctioning, the ladder gave way. I fell about 20-30 feet to the concrete floor next to the lift where the vehicles were being serviced and my face hit the edge of the lift. I was very fortunate that the lift was all the way down, otherwise I might not be around to write this book. The bottom of my lip and chin were all mashed up and my left knee was shattered. All I remembered someone saying was: "Don't touch him."

Four days later I woke up in a hospital bed. When I came to, I heard sounds seemingly coming from far away.

Someone said, "It looks like he is going to make it."

There were all kinds of tubes and wires attached to me. It was like a bad dream. There were nurses and doctors around my bedside. I tried to sit up but my entire upper body seemed quite heavy. I realized that I could not lift my head, I could not speak nor could I see clearly. There were stitches from my lower lip to under my chin.

The nurse informed me that my family was there. She cranked up the bed and said, "Your mother is here from Wisconsin to see you."

It was the very first time I got a glimpse of my mother in almost twenty years. She held my hands and spoke to me. What she said I did not know but she had a wonderful smile on her face. Then I drifted to sleep; I guess that was from all the medication given to me.

Subsequently, when I awoke again, my face felt very stiff and my hands were strapped to the bed, for what reason I did not know at the time. When I looked at my hands they were dirty with grease and oil. I assumed that was the reason they were tied. The nurse informed me that I had a major fall and they had to keep a close look on me. She told me that the doctor would be in to explain certain things to me.

I kept looking around for my mother.

The nurse left the room.

The following day this doctor entered the room and gave his name, which I don't recall. He mentioned that he was the surgeon who restructured the lower part of my face. He said that it was healing nicely. My heart was beating so hard I thought it would burst. He then took out a small mirror from a pocket on his white overall and handed it to me. My eyes were almost closed but the little I saw, my face was as large as a basketball. I cried and turned my face away from him.

Through the night my mind was troubled with many things. I was worried that all the hard work I had put into myself in terms of my food regimen and the benefits gained would now be lost. Denise visited me almost every other day to see how I was doing. I could not speak because of the stitches so I communicated with hand signals. Re also came to see me a few times.

While I was still at the hospital, an investigator came a few times to obtain evidence on what had happened. As I mentioned, I could not speak and after a while it became rather annoying so I would make signs trying to let them know that I would speak to him when I got out of there.

They shook their heads and left.

From the uniforms, I was able to tell that it was the same hospital I had spent most of my years with the sickle cell. After a few days I was moved to another ward. I had trouble walking and I was given physical therapy to improve this impediment. There was some concern about how I would manage when I was released from the hospital. Re extended an offer for me to stay with them until I was fully recovered. Some of the workers would come to see me on their way home from work and they would provide valuable advice to me. They advised me that I should not sign any documents. I was not interested in any of those things. My only concern was to go home, which I had not seen for some weeks.

On my release from the hospital, I was taken to Re's residence where I spent a week because all my doctors were in that county. Once again I was faced with more troubles. Michael, my son, had some medical problems. When I got out of the hospital, Denise informed me and sought my opinion before taking action. It was good that she waited.

Now, during these last few weeks, I had not eaten the way I should. Most of my food was liquids because I could not chew. There was news that I could not work at that dealer anymore because I created a problem for the company. Apparently, there was some kind of safety violation and attorneys were involved. The attorney who represented my interest inquired whether I wanted to return to work.

I responded with a resounding "No."

Now, apart from the injury I suffered, the company had stopped paying me. When I got out of the hospital I went on disability for about two years. With all this events taking place, my health was fading. This was because I could not maintain my eating habits and also, because of the amount of additional stress I was subjected to. Whereas before it was basically a mental struggle, it had now become a physical struggle also. I now had a broken body and a disease to contend with. I was not sure in what direction I should go at that time. One day I asked my girlfriend to take me to my former workplace and on the way there I thought about what I should say. I had to start somewhere.

I was half of a man. I had a busted knee and a mouth that was not functioning properly, so I didn't have enough weapons to work with. Although some of the workers were happy to see me, the owners were not. Some said that I should not sue the company. I listened to all their comments and when I was finished with the workers I went and sat with both the owner and manager. They realized that my injuries were severe. We discussed certain matters; we agreed on some and disagreed on others. I informed them that I did not know when I could return to work. I secured my equipment until I was able to remove them. I must tell you that the owners were not happy, as there was a suit against the company for negligence and use of improper equipment.

The matter took years in court and with that came a lot of stress such as medical bills and loss of work. There were also heated words that I was not welcomed on the property anymore. My attorney inquired whether I wished to return to work because they could not stop me from working there. However, after months of thinking about it, I decided that I did not want to return to work because there were too many unpleasant feelings. I waited until I was well enough to collect my equipment.

During all this time I was on soft food and liquids. This took me away from my new eating habits. My lower gum was mostly affected. Sometimes I would bite down on something that was a bit too hard and I this would cause my mouth to be in so much pain and my gum would bleed. When this happened, I would apply a hot compress to my chin and rinse my mouth with warm salted water. This went on a few days so during those times I could only drink warm liquids because my mouth was very numb, especially during the winter when it was cold. To this day I still have this problem but I have learned to live with it.

I needed to get back on track with my regular eating habits. One day I recalled that the wife of my grandfather on my mother's side had dentures. She only used them to chew meat and this was not often. She usually ate soft foods. One of the things she would do was to soak bread in buttermilk and eat it; she also crushed yams, potatoes and cooked vegetables and ate that. I eventually found a way to prepare my soft food or gum food, as I called it.

Foods need to be digested properly and to achieve that the food has to be well masticated with my saliva because the liquid has to travel to the liver, down to the bile where it has to go to the blood for inspection. Some of the foods that were important in my regimen, as I stated earlier, were garlic clove and red onion. Since I had difficulty in chewing foods, I had to devise a way to get the allicin extract from the garlic. The idea I came up with was to wrap three cloves of garlic in a piece of cloth, crush them, dip the cloth in a cup of warm water and suck on the soaked cloth so as to get as much liquid from the garlic as I could. It was very important to get the nutrient into the cells.

Garlic is a very important herb in any health problem because it contains an ingredient called allicin in which the nutrient is located. It has many anti-properties that will be absorbed into the tissue, the glands and the secretions in the body and destroy all the unwanted invaders that were attacking the body and, at the same time, it will heal and strengthen the body. It is one of the most unique herbs that could be used in any illness—anything from a cold, flu, lung problems to viruses of all kinds.

I persisted with the soft foods and my health improved considerably. It took a lot of determination but my goal was to take it to the end wherever that was. The year 1982 was a very tough time for me, having to deal with my son Michael's handicap, which I will not go into now.

During this period Denise's relatives thought that I needed someone to take care of me because of my chronic health problem and also, the latest injury. Well, little did they know that I had been doing this all of my life. My brothers and sisters and I were taught by our parents that it was important to take care of ourselves and I had learned that quite well. So the suggestion came up that it was a good time for Denise and I to marry. I was not listening because I did not want to go down that road. I had numerous problems and any talk of marriage at that time, I thought, would turn my whole life upside down. My few friends also did not think it was a good idea. However, her relatives were jumping for joy. I needed time to think about this.

Any time I went to her aunt's house, the aunt would put the question to me, "When are you getting married?"

I used to say to her, "I am thinking about it."

And she would say, "Don't take too long."

This went on for months. It weighed very heavily on my mind; when I thought about all the complications with living under the same roof with someone else, in my view that would be a huge step for me to take. I felt that there were more important things for me to take care of.

Around this time also, I had trouble getting around. I went to the doctors for therapy twice a week. I also had to concentrate on preventing any further damage to my organs and cells from the medication I was taking. I was advised by the doctors that I had no other choice but to take them so that my injuries could heal and also to get rid of the infection in my body. I did not fight with them on this issue. However, since I could not eat solid foods I drank bottled juice. Now, carrot juice tasted horrible to me but the health food store in my town did not carry any other juice. The juice was sold in glass bottles and this was one good feature about it.

My mouth constantly reeked of medication. One of the things that helped me a lot, which I mentioned earlier, was garlic. The other plant was the aloe vera, which I used on a neighbor's daughter who had a boil on a particular part of her body and I saw firsthand the wonders of this plant. I would go to the nursery and buy an aloe vera plant in a pot and take it home. I stripped the leaves of its gel and juice, added it to fresh juices and drank that mixture. Now, the taste was unbelievably bitter and that bitter taste stayed in my mouth for hours. Although I used sweet stuff to change the taste, as soon as the sweetness wore off, that acrid taste returned. The aloe vera was not only healing my mouth but also healing my body by ridding it of the poison from the medication; it brought my body into an alkaline state and cleaned my colon, the blood and the blood platelets.

In spite of these efforts, the accident set me back a long way. There were times when I wanted to quit. Also, when I looked all around and saw persons who looked healthy I would ask myself, "Why can't I be like them? Enjoying life?" I observed the smiles on the faces of persons around me and longed to be in their positions. Whenever I saw someone who looked unhappy I would ask, "Sir" or "Madam, why are you not happy?"

They would respond, "What is there to be happy about? I don't have the nice house or the fancy car."

And I would respond, "You have the greatest gift that one could have and that is life."

They would look at me as though I was crazy. Yes, I was sick but I was not crazy. When I thought about all the wonders of life around me that is what gave me the strength and the motivation to go on. These were the things that kept me fighting to live.

Another important lesson I learned was to take one day at a time. Many nights in my bedroom, the moon would spend a lot of time in that area and I would stare at it and wondered about the mythical man on the moon until it disappeared between the clouds. Then daylight would come, the next day would appear and the struggle would begin all over again.

No illness such as sickle cell disease is easy to overcome; it is a continual battle each and every day. It seemed as though life was getting tougher and tougher, in my case I had all these hurtles to climb over. Then I would get to the wall and all I could see was another wall. Deep down inside I knew that some day I would be over those walls but how exactly I did not know because I was only taking one day at a time.

Well, the sentence of five years in which I had to live was dispensed. It had come and gone and I am still here decades later. No one expected me to get this far in life with the sickle cell disease.

I know that it was only by the Grace of the Almighty and my insight to change my lifestyle that kept me going all through these years. By understanding His health laws that we so often neglect each day of our lives, and adopting them, I was able to survive.

As I look back, I recognize that the fear that physicians put in our minds could affect us for the rest of our lives. I have seen so many deaths that could have been avoided if only those persons had come to the realization and made the link between health and eating habits, as I had. In my case, all the doctors that I had seen about my health condition had all concluded that my time was running out and that I had only five more years to live. Being able to write this book thirty-two years later is evidence that I had proved them wrong and overcame this challenge.

One of the doctors I used to visit for treatment, concerning my health, had retired and moved to Barbados. He died later on.

OBSERVING THE LAWS OF NATURE

I am not sure whether anyone else with this type of disease has overcome it even today, where there have been so many improvements in the medical field. However, medical experts have not yet been able to conquer this disease that is plaguing many persons in this land and elsewhere. I am not even certain that a cure will ever be found for all these types of illnesses that are afflicting mankind because of our disobedience to the laws of nature.

The year is 1983. I was hearing from all sides that I should marry Denise, but I still was resisting as I did not think that I was ready for that new life. I also worried that I may die suddenly and leave this young girl a widow to raise a young child on her own. However, she and her relatives were not concerned about this; they said that was part of life. I, on the other hand, felt this was not what I wanted for my son. It was my wish that he would have a father to grow up with, especially because of his health concern so this was something constantly on my mind. Everywhere I turned the family was on my case about marriage. It was as though I could not catch my breath. My greatest fear was having my life turned upside down and coexisting with others in close proximity. As I said earlier, I was accustomed to my life one way and now it was going to change for the better or worse.

Since Denise was a Catholic, the family wanted her to be married in a Catholic church so we made an appointment to see the priest in the area that she lived. The date of the wedding was set. The appointment was in the evening and when we sat down, the first thing the priest asked me was, "Are you Catholic?"

I said, "No."

We were then informed that he could not marry us. We got up to leave but Denise asked to speak to him alone. I left the room. When she came out, she mentioned that he would speak to the Diocese in Philadelphia and get back to her. The family was influential members of that church and this was instrumental in us being married there. I subsequently had a few choice words with the priest, which I cannot relate here; but they were not nice. However, that was a long time ago and all is forgiven and forgotten.

About a month later we received permission to be married at this large church. Everyone was excited about the wedding. I did not have many persons to invite; I could count them on one hand, but Denise wanted to invite everyone she knew. While all the preparations were taking place I removed myself as I had fallen ill once again. I was not working, as there was a conflict with me going back to work. Somehow, all this stress was too much for me to handle.

I was rushed to the doctor's office as I did not want to return to the hospital. Everyone was concerned that I would be hospitalized. My blood pressure went through the roof; my heart rate was down to about fifty-three beats per minute. The doctors were quite worried about many things especially given the history of my health. However, I took the doctor's advice and got a lot of rest and went back on my food regimen.

I was grappling with a major concern; I could not get the proper fiber intake. Remember, in those early days there was no great support in this part of the east coast. The health stores were small and the managers or owners did not know much about nutrition. In fact, I had more stuff in my kitchen than some of the stores carried. Some of them were called herb stores and they had a few jars of bulk herbs and in most cases the ones they had were those I did not need. I would travel far and wide to locate a particular product and when I asked a question they did not know the answer so it was not easy for me to obtain the information or the products that I needed.

You may want to know why fiber? Why it was that important? Why I could not obtain it from the pharmacy or the grocery, or why I did not get the fiber necessary from all the raw food I was eating? Well those are very good questions. Yes, I was having a lot of roughage in my diet for the digestive system, and the small and large intestines. There is enough roughage in carrots but there is a complex compound of fiber in their unique form and it was difficult to obtain unless you had the proper method to extract the liquids. It also has a complex range of vitamins and minerals. Most of the fiber on the market does not have the nutrients in them; they are mostly processed fiber that has no benefit to the body. Everything I eat must have some benefit to the cell walls and major organs. I continued looking for solutions to overcome my health problems. At times it seemed as though there weren't any but my aim was not to give up or give in.

During my search I found a book written by Adele Davis called *Let's Eat Right To Keep Fit*. It contained some good points on vitamins but my objective was to maintain the kind of regimen I was on and that was the consumption of fruits and vegetables, which had brought me far. I had swallowed so many pills in the past that resulted in so many negative effects that I had to strive to build back the digestive structure and the saliva glands so vitamins were not my biggest fan at the time, unless it was in the form of liquids. Also, the vitamins were not of high quality so I preferred to stay away from them. I also found an old folk remedy book where the author used different kinds of herbal treatments, baths and enemas to heal people but there was no treatment to help sickle cell patients. The book had some fantastic information that could be put to use. These remedies were explained in a very simple manner. Once in a while I would come across a news clipping or articles in a *New England Journal* about sickle cell anemia but nothing concrete that could help me find the cure for this disease.

My greatest enemy was myself; struggling to overcome the everyday battle with myself. The wedding day was approaching quickly. I did not know what would be the outcome but in the meantime David, Darrell and Dexter were unhappy because they thought that the relationship would end once I got married. I had to assure them that I would always be around for them. I must confess that I broke that promise for a while but; as we all know, there are no guarantees in life. I would, however, receive these phone calls from Re advising me not to promise the kids I would be there for them because they usually waited around for me and then I didn't show up. When this happened, it was very difficult to win back their trust and confidence. They did not understand at the time that sometimes things do not work out the way they want them to but when I reminded them about my health issues, they would say to me, "We keep forgetting."

And they would ask, "Are you ever going to get better?"

I would respond, "Hopefully one day."

The time came for me to face life as a married man. I was given all the expert instructions on how to be happily married. Now, I had to throw all my attitudes and bad habits out the window. Well, it worked for a few months and then I was back to my old self. We were married in the fall of 1983; it was a beautiful wedding. I had a big surprise: my mother arrived late. She flew all day from Wisconsin because she had a few stopovers at other airports. She did not get there until late in the evening when everything was almost over, but it was a thrill for me because the last time my mother was in my presence was two years earlier when I was hospitalized for the accident and she visited me at the hospital. To see her for that special occasion was a joy and an inspiring moment for me. She was able to see her daughter-in-law and her grandson who, as I said earlier, is now deceased. It was an exciting time but for just a moment, because she had to catch an evening flight back to Wisconsin; the joy only lasted for a moment. She had the first cut of the cake that she took back with her. Her attendance was a huge surprise to me because no one alerted me that she was coming.

My cousin John was also there to support me; he was always there when I needed him. John my old friend and "brother" drove us to the church and reception hall. My friend Mike who introduced me to the doctor from the Philippines was also at my wedding to encourage me. It was a happy day for all of us. One of my younger sisters, Jean, flew across the Atlantic to be at my side. My brother Kelvin and sister Miriam made this beautiful three-tier wedding cake for me. It was fit for a prince. Everyone who knew about my illness was surprised about how well I looked. I had to explain that it was as a result of hard work and prayers; there was no other way to explain it.

I could not even explain it to my wife because I did not think she would understand.

It became very complicated for me to pursue my food regimen because having a young wife and a son in the same house, it was an uphill battle sometimes because they did not comprehend what I was trying to accomplish. They would remove everything from where I placed them. It did not matter how much I told them not to interfere with my stuff, they would remove them and place them elsewhere. These were some of anxious moments I went through and sometimes it was quite challenging. It was very difficult for me to deal with my health and marriage. It was not a good combination for me. It seemed that I was fighting a losing battle and it was getting harder for me to cope on a daily basis. I tried to deal with it by retreating to my bedroom and closing the door behind me. This is what I called being in a cracked shell. That is how I viewed myself, a cracked shell ready to explode in all directions as a result of all that was going on around me.

Two years have passed since the wedding. It has been a bit confusing as to which instruction or advice to follow. I know this may be a little difficult for you to understand but as a result of my illness all these years, I shunned many things because I was either too scared or I could not decide on what direction I should take. My life was like a seesaw; sometimes I was up and sometimes I was down. I could not follow directions and the reason for saying this is because I was to travel a different road in my struggle. Reading the *Bible* taught me a lot about life; it caused me to reflect on many things.

One night while I was watching a Boston television station a program came on called "The World Tomorrow" and there was a grey-haired old man talking about the *Bible* as I had never heard before. He was explaining things that made sense to me. The program lasted for about half an hour, at the end of which he offered some books at no cost. I took the phone number, called the number and requested those books. They took about a week to arrive and one thing I noticed was that they were very easy to read and understand. I gained a better insight into the principles of health and also the pitfalls when we do not follow those health laws.

I learned that ninety percent of all the food we eat is the wrong type and the body cannot use them and, therefore, it causes a chain reaction that leads to the breaking down of the organs. Then we are in no man's land. The blood is one of the first to be contaminated with the poison from the colon gases and its liquids. As I was discussing how I had a problem following instructions or heeding directions, take for instance whales and dolphins in the ocean, and even the elephants, they have a larger brain than the human beings, yet they cannot think, reason or make decisions on life. However, human beings who have a smaller brain than the whales, dolphins and elephants and are able to think, reason and make daily decisions on life sometimes act like those mammals and animals. I sometimes think that they do better than us by using their instincts.

I came to realize that I was not perfect; that my understanding was not yet complete and I knew that there was one greater than I and that some day all of us will gain that understanding and knowledge. But in the meantime I considered myself deficient in my understanding; what I call the missing dimension in knowledge of us human beings.

I have come a long way in my level of knowledge. I began to see the world differently and everything made sense to me now. Take for instance this disease I was fighting, I became aware of some of the causes. I also came to understand people with their health problems. I could look and see some of the causes. Bear in mind that many of our health problems are caused by what we do, say and eat. Our actions could cause a great deal of unhappiness, havoc, sickness and disease. One of the first things we do when we find out that something is wrong, is panic; before thinking, we make hasty decisions that take us downhill and when we get to the bottom, either it takes us a longer time to climb out or we don't get out at all. These are all things I have learned over the years. I must admit that I made many mistakes, some of which I did not fully understand. A man once told me that knowledge is power. Do I have power? No, but I have knowledge and understanding.

I paid greater attention to this gentleman on the television because he seemed to have an abundance of knowledge about the Great I Am and the problems in which mankind found themselves, which they could not solve because of lack of "true knowledge." This is why scientists are baffled, because true knowledge comes from above and only elected ones obtain this knowledge. He became my mentor. It was he who taught me the seven principles of what is required of a man in life. We will call him Herb. He was a man of wisdom; he lived a long and exciting life and passed away in his nineties years ago, but he left a legacy of knowledge for us to utilize in a booklet called *The Seven Laws of Success*. This booklet contains great principles for anyone who wants to achieve success in life.

With all that was going on around me: marriage, health issues, financial issues and the everyday struggle to overcome these battles, I was subpoena to attend court. This was in relation to the accident in 1975. I thought this matter was settled, but it was not over. My attorney kept trying to impress upon the company and the insurance company that it was because of the employer's negligence that I fell: the floor was greasy and no one was there to hold the ladder in place. I was put on the stand where I was cross-examined by the defense attorney about my health. He tried to blame the accident. He argued that as a result of my poor health I fell and blamed it on the company, which had an A-class background. He also claimed that I had no right to be in that part of the building. I kept looking at the attorney and would not respond. After a long frustrating half an hour on the stand, the judge asked me to step down. My attorney subsequently asked me to take the stand and answer the questions posed to me. After a tiresome day in court, I needed some good nourishing food to sustain me but there was none except for the regular stuff. This harrowing experience left me helpless for the rest of the week. I did not realize that you could be so drained from courthouse drama.

Well, the trial went on for about another year; it was a grueling experience. I felt as though I had committed a major crime. Although I was the victim of an accident, I felt that I was not treated well in the courtroom. The lawyers for the company had all the evidence. They engaged special agents to investigate the case. They had all my medical records for my chronic illness. They even went so far as to place the blame for the accident on the disease, but my attorney stood his ground. He even wanted to seek to move the case to another county because he felt that we would not have received a fair trial. Despite all these hiccups, we prevailed.

It might have been easier if the company had settled the matter out of court. The company was found to be negligent and was ordered to pay a moderate sum of money. This case took almost seven years to complete but it was worth it. After all these years, I still suffer with numbness in my lower lip and chin when the weather gets cold, but I have learned to live with it. Apparently one of the nerves was damaged by the surgery done on my lower lip and chin. I learned through the years that no one is perfect in this life; not even the doctors in whom so many put their faith and trust.

IN SEARCH OF A CURE

Through the years I had been hearing that the Native Americans had cures for any health problems so it was in my mind to investigate this, but was not sure how to go about it. I knew from history that the Native Americans in the west—the Sioux and the Dakota Indians—had lived in a place called Dells, Wisconsin and those Indians were still living up in those hills. In 1985 I had the opportunity to go west. I was on two missions: one, to see my mother whom I had not spent any time with since the early nineteen sixties. I saw her twice since that time: 1975 while I was hospitalized after the accident and in 1983 when I got married. This was going to be an exciting time for me. It was the fall of 1985; everything was arranged for my travel. Bear in mind that I had not seen any of my close family so this was a good beginning for me; and two, to attend a Fall Feast.

I was excited about this trip. My sister purchased a return ticket for me from New York to Wisconsin. Since I was not sure what kind of food was available there, I walked with mine own. I took green leaf cabbage, cauliflower and some of the other greens with me. One may wonder why my family did not accompany me since I was going to visit my mother. It was my intention to be on the move, hoping to find a cure for sickle cell, to visit my mother and to attend the Fall Festival at Dells, Wisconsin. I, therefore, did not know what kind of condition I would face.

My journey started in late September 1985. I took the train from Penn Station to New Jersey and then switched to another, which was a diesel engine at the time. Before we pulled out, some persons in my carriage were looking out the window because there was a bit of commotion with the train and switching the train on the right track to make sure everything was okay. The conductor blew the whistle for the train to take off after he was signaled to leave; so off we went. I could not afford a cabin with a bed and some of the other comforts but those of us who had regular seats received a small pillow and a small blanket because the nights were cold.

When we passed through some historic places, announcements were made and this made parts of the trip enjoyable. Once we got to Pennsylvania, they announced that we were entering the Horse Shoe Turn so everyone was trying to get a glimpse of it and to obtain a bit of history behind it. Some of the passengers were reaching across others to see this sight. I occupied a window seat and thus had full view. The scenery was very beautiful to look at with the lakes and the trees flashing by. As the leaves were beginning to fall, it looked like one of those forests in Lancelot as we journeyed through the scenic countryside. Whenever we went through a town the conductor would blow the whistle.

It was a long day and I was getting sleepy so I folded my pillow and got comfortable. We were in Pennsylvania so I thought by the time I awoke from my beauty nap, we would be entering Michigan but lo and behold, when I awoke, the gentleman next to me said, "You had a long, nice rest."

So I said, "We should be close to Michigan now."

I was surprised to hear him say, "We are still in Pennsylvania."

It was already nighttime so I went to the carriage where food was served and it was closed. Snack machines were available but I did not eat the contents of those machines. We traveled for hours on that train; I found out the next morning at breakfast that Pennsylvania is one of the longest states to cross over and this train was going non-stop to Chicago.

At dawn the next day, we were looking at that beautiful lake; it was so calm and still; it reminded me of when Moses was describing the creation when he said, "there was nothing; it was formless and empty and darkness was over the surface of this great depth." It was a large lake and then the dawn started appearing over huge expanse of water. It brought to mind what the earth might have really looked like at the very beginning of time; that must have been something spectacular to behold. The Creator took nothing and formed it into something; our human minds cannot even begin to comprehend that.

I learned a lot by traveling on the train, especially in the breakfast and dining room area. There were many people travelling to different parts of the country: some on business trips and some were on vacation. When I was asked where I was going and I told them to Wisconsin to visit my mother, they said, "That's a trip!"

I remember before I proceeded on the trip my mentor told me that in order to gain knowledge, you have to place yourself where people of that caliber reside. So I took advantage of that piece of advice by being at breakfast at seven-thirty in the morning. At this time there were congressmen, Senators and businessmen having breakfast and I would take notes. I leaned from the way they sat and how they used their cutlery. Oh yes, I was taking real notes. At times when I was asked what business I was into and I told them, I even got some of their names and addresses.

My buddy on the train was an older gentleman from Alabama whose name was Watkins; he was my sitting companion. He visited friends in New Jersey and was on his way home.

Well, our next stop was the Windy City—Chicago. There was an announcement that this was the train's last stop and everyone had to get off to catch another train if they were continuing on. Announcements were also made about destinations and the particular train to board. I became confused when the train pulled into the station; the massive crowd started running in all different directions. I had to push my way to retrieve my baggage before the train pulled off. As I reached for my bags, I was knocked over by the stampede. My suitcase went in one direction and the bag with the vegetables went in another. I found myself among these passengers trying to retrieve my vegetables. This was rather exhausting for me. I finally gave up. I inquired about how to get to the platform to board the train for Wisconsin and was directed there. Unfortunately, I missed the train that I was supposed to catch but it was not too long before I got another one.

The double-decker trains had just come into use; they were beautiful. I took a seat on the upper deck so that I could enjoy the countryside from above. Well, after all that excitement of running down my vegetables, I was very exhausted. It was a few hours ride but I was excited to get to Milwaukee. The train finally took off but when I saw where it was headed, I ran down to the lower deck to let the conductor know that I was on the wrong train. You see, a few persons said they were going to Milwaukee and I said Wisconsin and so I thought that I had boarded the wrong train.

However, the conductor allayed my fears when he said, "This train is going to Wisconsin."

Only then was my heart at ease. As the train roared passed the back of the suburbs, you were barely able to see what the cities really looked like from the outside but when we cleared the cities, we began to enjoy the lovely countryside. There were all these lush expanse of farmlands with huge cornfields and wheat fields. It was quite a picturesque sight to look at. As I said earlier, this trip was in the fall and so the landscape was really magnificent; I did not realize that so many beautiful areas existed in the country. Whenever I flew I missed the beauty of the land. I must say that travelling across country by train, there is a lot to see and to learn; it is very educational.

The sound of the intercom interrupted my thoughts. It was the conductor announcing that the next stop was Milwaukee, Wisconsin. I was very anxious so I got up and looked through the window to see if I could recognize my mother and sister, Princess. I had not seen my youngest sister since my wedding in 1983. As the train stopped I retrieved my suitcase and the rest of my vegetables.

I kept searching the faces of those gathered on the platform, but I saw no one whom I recognized; they must be late getting here, I thought to myself. I waited for about half an hour but no one showed up. I went in search for a payphone and called the number that was given to me. My mother was on the other end. I informed her that I had arrived and she told me that my sister had been there earlier and since she did not see me, she returned to work. I asked for the address and took a cab.

Although the driver did not know the area very well, in no time I was there. I was excited and so was my mother. She could not wait until I got out of the car before she started hugging and kissing me. It was one of the most joyful moments for her as well as for me, after so many years of not seeing my mother except for short sessions on two occasions; it was a sight to behold. Once we got into the house, she phoned my sister right away to let her know that I had finally arrived.

My mom prepared all these special dishes: fish, spinach, collared greens, rice and a lot of other delicious things. It was a banquet fit for a lost son. It was apparent that she had spent quite a long time preparing this special meal. She kept caressing my face like mothers do when they are happy or when their kids come to visit. I was her last boy, so I guess she still thought of me as her little boy. As I said before, my mother had only seen me briefly on two occasions over the past twenty-five years, so this was a very special day for her.

At one time there were even rumors that I was dead but my mother always knew in her heart that I was alive out there somewhere. She questioned me about all those missing years; there were no letters from me and no family member knew how to get in touch with me. She was anxious to know how I survived.

I said, "Mom, it is a long story. We will talk about it."

It was about half past two in the afternoon. My niece was just getting off the bus and my mother went down to the corner to meet her. I do not know whether my niece remembered me, but she was at my wedding three years before. She was about nine or ten years old now and was a very intelligent child. She kept telling me about her school and showed me her grades.

My sister finally got home about half past four in the afternoon. She had also seen me at my wedding also but before that, she had seen me since she was a child and as such she did not know much about me. I was considered the mysterious one in the family but it was a great family reunion. While my mother and sister were heating the food, my niece was setting the table. They placed all the food that I suspect my mother spent quite sometime preparing, on the table. I thought that other guests were expected, but I was wrong. My mom blessed the food and thanked the Great I Am for bringing me safely to Wisconsin and uniting me with part of my family.

She then said, "Go ahead and eat, son. There is plenty more here."

I hesitated to tell my mother that I could not eat the food she prepared for me. There was a big lump in my throat because I could not swallow. I did not want to hurt their feelings by refusing the meal so what I did, I ate everything else other than the meat. I then asked for the vegetables and was told that they were in the refrigerator. I made a salad to go with the meal. After dinner they brought out pastry and that was when I said, "Mom, could you hold the pastry?"

A while later I said, "Mom, I would like to tell you all something; I am a man who is dying slowly."

There was utter silence; you could have heard a pin dropped. She was confused.

My sister inquired, "What do you mean you are a dying man?"

I then related that I had a disease that I had been battling with for most of my life and it seemed to have the upper hand on me. They heard that the doctors had given up on me and had advised me in 1974 that I had five years to live. I explained that I was still fighting and seeking to find an answer. As a result of this, I was heading further west because I understood that the Native Americans in the Dells, Wisconsin had the answer for most of mankind's diseases.

Well, my mother thought I was crazy and that I did not know what I was talking about. She never heard of such a thing. She went further to say that there are other doctors who could heal my pains. She extended an invitation for me to stay with them but I told her I did not want to be a burden to anyone. I also reminded them that I had a new family that I had to take care of.

She was flabbergasted, "How could you take care of a family when you can't even take care of yourself?"

My response to her was, "Mom, time will tell."

I could see that Mom was hurt by what she had just heard. I kept reassuring her that everything would be all right.

I said, "I have come this far, how much further I will go, I don't know; all I could do is to keep on going until my time runs out."

I hugged my Mom and I told them I would see them in a few days; I also promised to call. My sister and I left; she followed behind me in her car for a short while since it was some distance from Milwaukee to the Dells.

The time was eleven o'clock at night. My sister followed me as far as a gas station; we hugged and then she turned around and left. I was in the middle of nowhere. As I looked around there was this country bar; the front area was lit up but the rear was quite dark. There was a jukebox playing country and western tunes. As I walked into the bar with the noise blaring and trying to get the cashier's attention, some big men who were about six or seven feet tall advanced towards me. I backed up to the doorway, threw my hands into the air and shouted out that I was from New York. They stopped advancing towards me; they bought me a drink and I told them about New York, the city that so many had heard about but never visited. I also let them know that I was on my way to the Dells but that I was lost. I was directed to go down the street, and then make a left turn. I handed the girl at the cash register a twenty-dollar bill for their drinks and I left. I must tell you that I was terrified of those men because I thought they were going to lift me bodily and throw me out of the bar. I followed the direction they gave me.

EXTREME COLD AT DELLS WISCONSIN

I realized that I was about ten minutes away from my destination. I got on the main road that was lined with stores; everything was closed. I did not have a place to stay since I did not make any hotel reservation. The night was dark and extremely cold. While driving along the street, I saw a payphone. There was also a hotel across from it called Black Hawk Hotel. I pulled up close to the payphone and took the receiver into the car so that I could make a phone call. I pulled a telephone directory attached to a long chain into the car and I went through the yellow pages searching for hotels in the area. I dialed the numbers to see if anyone would answer the phone at that time of night. I did not get a response.

Within half an hour my feet and fingers began to get numb, as the heater in the small car was not functioning properly. I kept my jacket buttoned all the way up, wondering what my next move would be. I uttered a small prayer and asked myself the question: "What am I doing here in this freezing weather with no proper winter gear?"

I decided to drive the car across the street to the hotel. I kept the headlights on and through the curtain I could see someone sitting on the couch in the lobby, apparently asleep. I knocked on the door but I saw no movement. I banged harder; the gentleman got up, walked to the door, moved the curtain and waved to me, indicating that there was no more room and he went back to the couch. By this time I was freezing. I drove back across the street next to the phone booth. I was sleepy; I cracked the window a little so that the toxic fumes from the car's exhaust would not affect me.

Now, I was beginning to get cramps in my legs. I once again decided to go back to the hotel and knock on the door. I thought about what I would say to this guy when he woke up because I knew he would be mad. Of course, as I knocked on the door he got up, opened the door and yelled at me, "I told you there is no room."

By this time I had placed one foot in the doorway to make it difficult for him to shut the door. I said, "Sir, I just want to ask you a question."

"What?" he shouted.

And I asked, "Is there any place you know around here that I could spend the night?" Because of the amount of noise he made earlier, a woman got up and came to the door and she asked me to come in.

That lady saved my life that night because I might have frozen to death. My fingers were stiff and could not move; my feet were numb and my face felt like rock. I stood in that office for about five minutes and felt the heat on my face. It was as though snow was on my body and the heat was melting it. I could not have asked for a better gift. I would have given whatever valuables I had on me that night to keep warm.

While the gentleman was still fussing, the lady said, "Wait a minute, I might know a place where you could spend the night."

Boy, you should have seen my face. It lit up like a bright light glowing in the dark.

She asked, "Are you driving?"

I answered, "Yes."

She then directed me to go out the door, turn left down the driveway and go down to the end and made another left and I would see a light.

"It's right there."

I followed the directions and as I pulled up, the light was on, and there was a gentleman waiting for me. I informed him that the lady at the Black Hawk Hotel sent me.

He said, "You mean my sister-in-law." Then he said, "You are lucky; someone cancelled the booking at the last minute."

I stayed in a cabin. There were several of them. Each family had their own unit. I signed the register, paid for my stay, which was eight days and the gentleman handed me the keys and directed me to the cabin. I parked the car under the carport, took out my baggage and went to the unit. I opened the door and felt the cold wind against my body. I turned on the light and there was a small heater blowing cold air. I was too tired to make a fuss about it. That night I went to bed with all my clothes just so that I could keep warm. The jacket had a hood, which I pulled over my head. I did not have any gloves so I placed my hands in my pockets. Through the course of the early morning I could hear the wind swirling around outside. There were times I wanted to go to the bathroom, but I refused to move from the spot where I lay because I wanted it to remain warm. It was a rough night for me.

The following morning I went to the office and informed them about my experience with the lack of heat; they apologized for that situation and promised to take care of the problem. Luckily for me there was hot water so I sponged off real quickly and put my undershirt back on because it was much warmer than those in the suitcase. As cold as it was, I had to change my underpants because my parents used to tell us never wear dirty underwear just in case we fell ill and someone had to come to our aid. Well, I was partially clean and ready to face the day.

I inquired about breakfast and was sent up the street on the left hand side. Well, it seemed as though it was the only place in Dells, Wisconsin where breakfast was served. The lines were stretched around the corner and the cars were lined up blocks waiting to get in the parking lot. I had to wait quite a while to be seated. It was difficult to obtain a seat for one person so I shared a table with a family of three. By the time the waitress got to our table, it was almost time for me to leave so I decided on a light breakfast.

As I sat there and looked around, it was quite amazing to see what people were ordering. I remember the couple across from where I sat ordered chocolate shake with two scoops of vanilla ice-cream, two eggs with bacon and ham, coffee and a side order of fried potatoes. When the waitress stepped over to me she apologized for the long wait. I browsed through the menu and could not find anything that was acceptable to me except juices and teas.

I ordered a large glass of freshly squeezed orange juice and two slices of plain, toasted rye bread.

She took one look at me and said, "You can't get no freshly squeezed orange juice and you can't get no rye bread." And then she walked over to the cook in the kitchen and said, "There is a man here from up North who wants freshly squeezed orange juice and toasted rye-bread."

By this time all eyes were on me in the diner. One of the cooks came out to see who was this man making such a request.

He walked over to the table and asked, "What is rye-bread?"

I was not in the mood to go through an explanation.

He then said, "I only have white bread and the regular orange juice."

I ordered the juice, drank it and left.

I was already late for the feast in the morning. On the second day I began to investigate the story about the Dells' Native Americans. I was introduced to a gentleman who was the captain on the riverboat that traveled up river. On the third day, I was anxious to take that trip. The captain informed me that at that time of the season they did not go up river because it was cold and could be very windy or the waters could be frozen at certain areas, but this was my only chance to go. I do not recall how much it cost to travel up there but cost was not an issue for me. It was one of the reasons I made all the plans to go to Dells, Wisconsin.

During this time I was so busy that I forgot to call my mom to let her know that I was okay. They kept calling the phone number I had given them to contact me. When I returned to my cabin, I found out that there were a few messages left for me to call them as soon as possible. So I asked to use the telephone in the office to call my mother who wanted to know how I was doing and when I would be returning. I told her I would be back on the evening after I had finished with some work that I had volunteered to do. The next call I received was from my wife who also wanted to know if I was okay and enjoying myself. I could not tell her what was going on. I just said to her that everything was fine and I that I would be home soon. Even though things were not going well for me, I could not let her worry.

Well, the time had come for the trip up river. On the fourth day, the boat was gassed up and ready to go. The time planned for leaving was half past twelve in the afternoon. The sun was out; it was about fifty degrees that day; we boarded the boat and headed up river. Let me pause here for a moment. It reminded me of a movie I had seen once with Humphrey Bogart and Katharine Hepburn (I don't remember the name of the movie, but it was one where he had an old boat trying to outfox the Germans in an African river). We continued up river with the captain making all these twists and turns because of all the bends in the river. It was very beautiful scenery; there were larva rocks, some of them like little islands. The captain gave us some of the history of the river and the trades with the Native Americans. They took fur pelts and other animal skins down to the depot to trade for food to take back to their camps. I have not seen so much hidden beauty as in the wilderness high up in the Wisconsin upper river.

After some time, the captain finally announced, "We are here!"

The boat pulled up alongside an old jetty; he told us that we had half an hour. I got out the boat; it was quite cold. There was an old trail ahead of me and I hurried along it to see what I could find. There were many tall pine trees in the area. I was hoping to find a tepee but as far as my eyes could see it was only more trees ahead and water. Half an hour was not enough time to conduct any search. I did not even know what to look for. I guess I was hoping to meet someone there to ask questions or obtain information about the Native Americans living in the upper region of the Dells.

A had a lot of excitement planning this trip, but it was becoming a bit of a disappointment for me. However, I always tried to take negative things in life and turn them into positives. I thought about the beauty that I saw there and then I thought about the creation and the beautiful things that life had to offer. When we returned from that trip up the river, I was told to try down river. But from speaking to some of the elderly residents, I was informed that there was nothing interesting down river and that all the history was in the upper Dells.

I elected to visit some of the dairy farms as some of my colleagues had asked me to bring back some aged cheese for them since Wisconsin was the home of aged cheese. This country road I took had some of the most magnificent trees I had ever seen. The area looked quite picturesque. Although it was late fall, the leaves had not completely fallen off the trees. I understand that those persons who could afford to leave there in the winter had already left by the end of September and headed for Florida or somewhere warm.

Now at this farmhouse there were these large containers where the milk was poured from; the milk went through different stages where it was constantly turned and left to set for a period of time to make that special brand of cheese. The process for making the aged cheeses was very interesting. I also had the opportunity to sample the different kinds of aged cheese, which were served with crackers.

That evening I decided to visit my mom in Milwaukee; I knew it was a long ride. I left the Dells around four o'clock in the afternoon. However, my sister had left a message that if I was planning to visit I should not bother to do so because there was a storm heading that way. I did not go back to the cabin because I was closer to the entrance to the highway than my cabin. I headed to Milwaukee to spend the night with the intention to leave early the following morning to return to the Dells.

All of a sudden the clouds gave way and there was pouring rain. At times visibility was so poor that I had to drive with great caution. The windows were fogging up and the heat in the car was not working well but with all the odds I got safely to somewhere in Milwaukee. I found a payphone and called my sister.

I said to her, "Guess what? I am a few blocks from the house but I can't find it."

She said to me, "Didn't you get my message?"

Of course, I asked, "What message?"

I then informed her that I was out all day and did not return to the cabin. I gave her an indication of where I was located and she gave me directions to the residence. Well, mom was quite happy to see me so once again it was a delightful time for my mom, my sister and me. The meals were different this time around. She cooked food which had no life but I learned to be modest when I am in someone's home or when I am on the road travelling.

You may remember a few pages back when I went to the only large restaurant in town, which accommodated hundreds of people at that time. I learned that everyone didn't know about the quality of food and its purpose for life. When I saw what people ate for food, it was no wonder that many died prematurely or were struggling with illness, and that includes me also. I understood why I had this type of disease, the sickle cell or traits. I could not blame anyone at all. It was merely a case that I did not know way back then what I discovered years ago. If I go back as far as I could remember, I ate some obnoxious things that are called food. There are certain foods that mankind should not eat, but some of us eat them anyway. I now have a better understanding about this aspect of life. It is important that we use wisdom in everything we do. I learned to give honor to the Great One above for all things.

My trip to Wisconsin Dells was not in vain. It was an education for me. My mother did not understand the purpose of the food was for my health at that time. She was honoring me; instead I should have been the one honoring her. I realized that it takes humility to honor and I did not have humility. That was the greatest lesson I learned over the years: how to grow in humility.

I returned to the Dells the following day, stayed there for a few more days then I returned to Milwaukee, spent a few hours with mom until my sister took me back to the train station to head back to New York. I had a lot of work to do. I found out that it was not just the sickness but I also had to learn many things about myself.

What is the point in being ill, recovering from that illness and remaining the same joker in the deck? When you are ill and you overcome that illness you should be thankful; you should have a compassionate heart for others. You should have love for one another. You should be more grateful in everything you do like praying for others when they are sick instead of thinking about yourself. Why don't you think about someone who has more health problems than you? In doing so, one could reap great benefits as I did in past years.

When I look at the scenery and the beauty of this great master plan that has been given to us we sure made a mess of it. In the breakfast cart while traveling back to New York, I sat and observed things around me, as I usually did. Sometimes people would ask if they could sit with me and I would say, yes. On this return trip I noticed the way people ate; they ate as though they were hungry so they put large chunks of food into their mouths and spoke at the same time. At times they would be choking; then they would have some of the water from the glass that had been put before them.

When I looked at the quality of food they served and the quality of food they ate for breakfast, this is what I saw: eggs, fried, boiled or easy over; light sausages, bacon, ham, potatoes fried in some grease, hash brown, toasted white bread or whole wheat bread with butter along with orange juice, cow's milk or black coffee with sweet and low. Now, this type of breakfast alone will cause major health problems later down the road. There is nothing in such a breakfast that would sustain life in its energy force. Not only that, the food would take about eight hours to get through the stomach and the small intestine where sometime later it will enter the large colon and continue poisoning the system.

I finally arrived home, exhausted from the trip. All I wanted to do was sleep and get back to everyday living. My wife was eager to know everything that happened out there. She commented that I looked as though I was starving. I informed her that there was not a lot of prepared food available that I could eat.

My son would ask, "Mom what happened to dad?"

She would respond by saying, "Your father is tired from his trip; let him rest."

After I slept for a couple of days it was as though my body had a hunger and thirst for the foods and fruits I had not eaten for ten days so I doubled up on my special foods, eating things I like most: garlic cloves, carrots, scallion, cauliflower, cucumber and many other greens. I was back on my feet not too long after that and was ready for another adventure.

Remember, my goal was to find a cure or some type of treatment for sickle cell and, therefore, I intended to follow whatever leads I got. My sight was much wider spread because I had the taste of the trail, which was not an easy one. So I decided to return to Wisconsin one more time. I felt that there were some things I did not see or which I overlooked. I made arrangements to stay at the same place. I booked early so that I would not encounter any of the problems I had the last time. I worked hard and saved some extra money for my trip.

I loved to travel in the fall because less people are on vacation then. I realized that mostly business people traveled at that time of the year so airports and train stations were less crowded. My mentor taught me this lesson. Also, the fares are lower at that time of the year so it was my favorite time to travel, but this time I was going by air. My wife did not like me going off on these crazy adventures following these fall flowers, but I had a mission to accomplish and that was to discover the cure for sickle cell.

That is all I was living for at that time. I was putting all my energy into this goal. I did not understand many things about the True Source who said to "cast all your burdens on Him." I did not understand that faith is the substance of all things and I did not have this faith so I was looking to myself and trying to unravel a mystery. I did not have the slightest idea what I was doing until I started to read the Great Book that the Great I Am gave to mankind to study and understand the human body.

I returned to Wisconsin in the fall of 1986, late in October. It was colder than my previous trip. I flew from MacArthur Airport, Long Island to Chicago then to Madison, Wisconsin. My flight was delayed. I caught another flight to St. Louis and connected to Madison. I had already given the hotel my flight information and the time I would get there, so I called the hotel desk and provided the new information. They assured me that everything would be fine whatever time I got there. The flight from St. Louis departed about half past nine in the evening. Now, I left my hometown, Long Island, at seven o'clock in the morning and at nine o'clock in the evening I still had not arrived at my destination. I touched down in Madison, Wisconsin at eleven o'clock. It was a small airport; most of the shops were closed because all flights had already come in except this last flight from St. Louis.

I stepped off the plane; everyone was running to the baggage area to collect their luggage. I inquired about car rentals and was directed to the area. I was running to catch the car rental open; as I turned around, the airport was in darkness. The rental place was about to close. I yelled at the guy to wait because I needed a car. I was quite lucky because it was the only car left on the lot. I signed the contract; I was given directions and I left. As I departed from the airport it started to rain. By the time I got onto the highway it was raining heavily; the windows were fogging up and visibility was very poor. I kept driving at a minimum speed because I did not know that part of the country; I was indeed very cautious. However, while traveling on the highway, there was a long flat bed truck with very poor lights approaching me. It was doing about 70 miles per hour on this wet highway. I thought it had passed me but as I was continuing to get closer to the curb I kept blowing my horn but apparently the driver could not hear me. Finally, I was able to get the car on the edge of the median just before the car went down into the ditch. It was a close call for me that October night.

I got to the resort at about one o'clock in the morning and the office was closed. I had my room number so I proceeded to the cabin. I got to the room, opened the door, put my bags on the floor and turned the light switch on. Guess what? There was a couple asleep on the bed. I woke them up to let them know that they were in the wrong cabin.

The man said to me in a menacing way, "You better get out of here!"

I was not about to argue with them at that time in the morning; I just took my stuff and put them back in the car and pulled the car under the carport to face a cold night. I was tired from traveling all day and then when I got to my destination, things didn't work out for me although I had made all the necessary phone calls to ensure that I did not run into the kind of problems I faced the last time. I had warmer clothing this time but when it is this cold, if you are not in a well-heated place, you would still feel the cold. The car was not the most comfortable place to sleep but I did the best I could that night.

The next morning, I went to the office and complained about their breach of our oral agreement. They apologized for the mix up. A gentleman explained that a note was left in the office for me to take the other cabin. I do not have to tell you how very upset I was. I made him aware that I had to sleep in my car and that it was very cold; he kept apologizing. I vowed that I would not conduct business with them again. I once again stayed there for eight days.

I had signed up to assist parking of the vehicles at the feast site. It was so cold at five o'clock in the morning at the site and there was no protection from the wind. It was so cold that coffee was brought out for those of us who were assisting with parking. Since I did not drink coffee, when they brought me a cup I took off my gloves and put my fingers inside the coffee to warm them up. This is how I managed to get rid of the numbness in them. By the time the shift changed at nine o'clock in the morning, I was almost frozen. It is a time in which I saw men struggle to stay warm. It did not matter how many layers of clothing I had on, I still felt the cold in my bones. We were told that this cold air came off the great lakes. The two days I signed up for was enough for me, although at the end of the day I had to go to my cabin at nights and sleep in a cold room. This was really too much for me to bear.

One day I decided to visit my mother to get some sleep. It was about a two to three hours drive to Milwaukee, depending on the time I left the Dells, Wisconsin. It was refreshing to sleep on my sister's waterbed although it was a bit uncomfortable. I spent one night and was all refreshed for the next day's ride back to the

Dells, where I was scheduled to meet a few people who had invited me to join them deep in the Wisconsin woods to spend a day.

We drove for a while and walked the rest of the way. I kept asking myself, "Where are we going?" It seemed like there was no end. I marked certain trees as we went along; there were many winter critters around. I knew that there were no bears in the woods at that time as they were already hibernating in the caves for the winter.

We finally got to our destination; a few of the persons in the group had been there before. There was a large cabin, which could accommodate about twenty-five persons. The food that the group had in their possession was peanut butter, white bread, roast beef, hot dogs, the Wisconsin aged cheese, mustard, canned soup, water, soda, apple juice, orange juice and potato chips. There were about twelve of us in the cabin. Of course, I could not eat any of the food. For some reason the temperature dropped in the woods and our food had all been consumed. All that was left was the apple juice; they had consumed all the sodas and orange juice. There was a small fire going; we all huddled together as the penguins up in the Arctic to stay warm. The apple juice was freezing up and was too cold to drink. Some of us started to use our survival skills to get through the time. We poured all the apple juice into a pot and put it on the wood fire until it came to a boil and then we passed it around with each person taking small sips at a time, because we only had so much to go around.

I noticed that when it was my turn to drink they were so generous to allow me to have more than the rest of them because I did not have anything to eat. I could not eat the type of food they brought along. I also noticed that the hot apple juice was creating warmth in my body. My head got hot and my feet became warm and the numbness in my toes was disappearing. When the juice started to cool, we would heat it up again. Before long, everyone was feeling a bit warmer. Who would have thought that hot apple juice would have eased some of our pain in a cold wood cabin in the forest of Wisconsin? I would not have believed if I had not been there myself to find out first hand.

While we were in that cabin many conversations on different topics kept our minds occupied and kept boredom at bay. We talked of places we would like to visit and where we had been. I listened most of the time since my main aim was to seek and obtain information and knowledge from all those around me. Some of them mentioned that the following year they would be heading to the west coast; some were going to Arizona and they talked about things that were of interest to me. So I decided there and then that the west coast and Arizona would be good places for me to visit to see what I could find.

THE ARIZONA DESERT

After I returned home I gave my decision further thought. I worked harder and saved for the trip the following year. I obtained all the information about Tucson, Arizona and also the cost of hotel accommodation for ten days. I made reservations at the Ramada Inn six months ahead. Arizona was known as one of the great places to visit during the winter months when the weather got really cold. Since I did most of my traveling during the fall, I felt that it would be a good place to visit and hopefully gather lots of information. Remember, throughout the sixties to the eighties there was no cure for this disease and I had been fighting this disease from the seventies. This was my third exploration trip and I was alone once again except for the One who was always there for me whenever I needed Him for answers.

In the fall of nineteen eighty-seven, I embarked on the trip to Tucson, Arizona for a period of ten days to explore and also attend a Feast site. It would be my first time in that part of the country. The scenery was magnificent with the kind of copper tone, gold colored mountains and different varieties of cactus everywhere. Some were as tall as palm trees.

Upon my arrival and as soon as I settled into my hotel room I went to the convention center and viewed all the Presidential pictures except one, and that was the first President of the United States who is not George Washington. There was a President before Mr. Washington, who was from Massachusetts. His name was John Hanson who served from Nov. 1781 to Nov. 1782. President Hanson established the Great Seal of the United States. George Washington was the first Constitutional President.

While I was there I heard about a museum in the desert that I was very excited to visit. I thought I had hit the jackpot so I got back to my hotel and made some phone calls. The person I spoke to stated that the tour starts at eight o'clock in the morning because of the hot weather. That night I could not sleep. The next morning, I dressed in short sleeve shirt, cool long pants and armed myself with some water and snacks in my shoulder bag. I arrived about seven in the morning waiting for the tour to begin. As soon as there were enough persons, the tour began and before I knew it, I was separated from the party.

Fasten your seatbelt because you are in for a treat. I got lost in a sizzling Arizona desert. When I caught myself, I was in no man's land.

I tried not to panic but everything around me looked the same. I was not worried about the snakes at that time of the day because I knew they were in some place cool and most of the critters only moved about at nights when it was cooler to hunt their prey. What I was worried about were scorpions and other deadly desert creatures.

I recalled then that when my grandfather and I were in the fields he would ask me, "What time is it?"

I would say, "Grandpa, I don't know."

He would say to me, "Look up at the sun and see where it is."

And I would respond, "I can't look at it."

Then he would look and he would say, "Twelve noon." He explained that when the sun was in the middle of the sky over your head it is high noon, but the problem was that I could not look directly at the sun; it was extremely hot out there in the desert. However, I shaded my eyes from the sun and estimated its distance; then I tried to locate east, west, north and south. I also tried to calculate the distance of my shadow between east and west. I also remembered my father would sit at the window and say, "See the moon, look at what is next to it; a star, and it is different from all the other stars; it is larger and it follows the moon south west."

I knew those were some of the signs I had to look for when the time came. I tried to remain positive but my throat was rather dry. I started to lose my stride. When the sun was at the back of my shoulders and neck, I knew that I was going in the wrong direction. The sun should be in front of my face and I should be heading west, to where the sun would set in the evening.

My greatest fear was being bitten, even an ant, because the poison could be deadly. I heard the sound of the birds and I tried to see where they were coming from. Little lizards ran past me or jumped across my path. My face, my hands and the rest of my body that was exposed to the sunrays started to burn. I thought of the cool hotel room I left behind. What would I have done for a cool drink of water or some melon or papaya juice?

All of a sudden, I thought I heard a noise like an engine of some sort. I thought my mind was playing tricks on me because there was some noise coming from the distance that seemed to be getting closer. Lo and behold, it was a jeep; the jeep passed me and stopped a short distance away. Nonetheless, I kept walking until I felt someone's hands around me; it took me a few seconds to realize that it was actually someone who was there holding me. This lady helped me into the jeep and while she was driving she said to me, "What are you doing? You could have died out here."

All this time I had not spoken a word because my throat was parched and I was afraid to open my mouth. She put a cold rag against my throat, neck and face. She was trying to keep me cool. We finally got to the place where I should have been in the first place, the museum. It resembled a tunnel and it was quite cool. I thought I was in paradise. As we continued there was water running in little streams. There were various species of the desert critters. She pointed out that lizard is one of the reptiles that could cause great harm when it bites. I saw some of the menacing looking rattlesnakes. Then as we proceeded along we came to where there were fossils in water. You could only observe them through the glass container in which they were stored. By now I was feeling a lot better. The lady asked me for my name and I told her who I was and what I was doing in Arizona. I informed her that I was dying and I was searching for a cure. She wanted to know what I was dying of and I told her I had sickle cell, which crippled my nervous system.

She explained that they usually drove a thirty-mile range searching for persons who may have wandered off. We eventually got to this wide-open space; there were steps leading upstairs. She asked me to wait there. She said, "Please don't move from here."

I responded, "Where would I go? I will be right here when you get back." I kept my word and stood there, not knowing what next to expect. There was no one coming or going from where she disappeared. I did not hear any voices, which would have indicated that someone else was around. I was tired from standing; my legs were still wobbly from the amount of walking I had done. I don't know how long she had gone, maybe half an hour or an hour, I really cannot say. While I was waiting, there was the sound of an explosion. I hit the floor and covered my ears. I thought the cave had just been dynamited but there were no rocks falling on me so I raised my head and looked around, everything was a blur; so I got up and there was a screen with an awesome display of the evolution of the planet earth was beginning. At first the screen was blank, then some color was introduced and it faded away. Then appearing on the screen was 7,000 years, 6,000 years, 5,000 years and so on. By the time 1,000 years flashed across the screen, planet earth's life form was showcased in all its beauty. I kept looking at the screen in awe. I heard another explosion coming from my right and this time I found myself in a stooping position. When I looked to my right, there was another screen way back in the corner. I really did not notice that that before. On that screen was a volcano erupting. It seemed so real as though the lava was spilling out from the screen and flowing towards me. I backed up a few steps.

Now, during all this time I had seen no one else. Apparently the lady who brought me to the museum and I were the only ones there. A little later she returned with a package in her hand. She asked where I was staying and I informed her that I was staying at the Ramada Inn. She drove me back to the hotel and held my hand as we entered the hotel. She inquired whether I was going to be all right.

I answered, "Yes."

She handed me the folder. She promised that she would return later. Now, this young lady was very attractive. She was about 5'2" and weighed about 100 to 105 pounds. Her hair was combed back; her hair and skin were as pretty as the color of the desert mountain with the sunset reflecting on it. This is about the best way I could describe her. I cannot say if she came back to the hotel to see me because I slept in my room for the next three days. I was over-fatigued, dehydrated and run down from the desert heat.

A few days later, I asked the desk clerk if there was a health food store in this area. He directed me to one a few blocks up the street. I was weak and tired and looked like burnt charcoal. When I get out in the heat, my skin began to burn. It was a sunny Sunday morning. I got there and saw people lined up on the sidewalk. I realized then that the store was closed and they were waiting for it to open. I joined the line. What I saw indicated to me that these people were dedicated to their health or were interested in health issues.

The store opened at eleven o'clock in the morning and the crowd rushed in. I, however, was in no hurry. After all, I still had a few days left, so time was on my side. I wanted to ensure that I did not miss anything. It was not a classy health food store. It was like an old country store; it was just what I was looking for because there may be something old which I may find interesting. I browsed around the produce section and found grapes, papaya, berries, nuts and seeds. I had to consume more of the organic juices because of the dehydration of my body. I knew from experience that the organic juices were more replenishing to the body, especially when it was injured. I normally crushed watermelons, papaya and grapes together like a soup. The watermelon produces more juices than the others due to the high content of water.

There were many little things in the health food store that I did not find in the stores in the New York area and other places. In one corner was a book section, not a large selection, but enough to stimulate my appetite. As I searched the shelves I found a book written by Jethro Kloss, called *Back to Eden*. It was written in 1938. I paid for the stuff and left the store.

I spent most of the rest of my time in my hotel room because I was avoiding the desert heat; it was much cooler there. Although I left the room at nights when the sun went down, it was still hot but there no sun rays to burn my skin. While in my room, I browsed through the book and the folder that my "angel" gave me. The folder contained pictures and information about the prehistoric dinosaurs and other reptiles and the millions of years they lived on this planet, other specific things about the earth and also the volcanic disturbance of the earth. It was very interesting stuff.

One night I picked up the book *Back to Eden*. Lo and behold, I read it from cover to cover that same night. The information it contained was like gold nuggets in the rocks. The more I read the book the more sense it made. Jethro Kloss was a very interesting man who ran a sanitarium to help sick persons and those who sought knowledge. He also knew a lot about farming. He had superior knowledge about herbs; he travelled the country from coast to coast helping people. He had a passion for the use of herbs, or what I refer to as understanding God's nature.

He also understood food, the right type of food that would heal the body when it was injured. He was also one of America's leaders in health and nutrition in respect of health problems.

I was astonished to know that there was someone who had such a wealth of wisdom about the human body. The information in that book helped me to understand that the food regimen I was practicing was not in vain. It also gave me hope and a new lease on life and the belief that I could overcome this disease. As a matter of fact, I believe that understanding the body, working hard and introducing the right type of minerals and the other elements that the body requires could overcome any disease that ails mankind.

For the next few days I spent most of my time at the health food store searching for new material and asking questions, but the persons at the store were not quite knowledgeable on the subject of health. They wanted to know where I got my information and I would say, "From 'The Great I Am.'" They would look puzzled. I purchased another small book called *Build Up With Foods That Alkaline and Heal* by Mrs. C. Hoggs. It talked about the use of carrot juice to build and alkalinize the body. As I found out, I was ahead of my time in respect of health issues. Juicing by hand method was something I had known about because I did not own a juicer nor did I know where to locate one.

Two of the greatest foods on the planet are the carrot and the lemon. They are both alkaline but one is a fruit and the other is a vegetable.

When both are put to the proper use they can offer tremendous benefits and are effective in bringing the body back to its natural state. Carrot juice is the only raw juice that I know that has three of the most important vitamins that fight off diseases and build the sick body back to its natural state, and these are vitamins A, C and G. Carrot will restore a weakened digestive system, repair the lungs and mucus membrane and all the glands that are affected by diseases, provided that these carrots are grown in the proper soil. Although foods may look alike, the difference is the soil in which they were grown. That makes the difference in foods.

I learned a lot in the ten days I spent in Tucson, Arizona. I came away with more information than I would ever receive from anywhere else. I did not see my "Angel" before I left nor did I find out her name, but I thank her and would always be grateful to her for taking me out of that scorching desert. If it were not for her I may not have been here to write this book. I only hope that whoever she was that in all things her joy may be made whole.

I wish to caution the readers of this book; whenever you go on any trip with a guide, do not for any reason believe that you know more than those who are there to guide you; follow all instructions given to you or the group, especially when you are not familiar with the territory. I thought I knew enough to venture out on my own. I was also anxious to get out and explore the desert of which I had little knowledge. Another warning, do not try to use my calculation because it would not work. You must possess great wisdom and experience in calculating the time of day without the use of proper instruments.

Well the time had come for me to head back home. I considered it a good trip and one that I really enjoyed. I arrived home with little souvenirs for my son and Denise that they always looked forward to.

Before you knew it, I was already planning for yet another trip; this time I decided to take my son who was seven years old at the time. I knew it would be a bit more burdensome but this is what I wanted to do. Well guess what? I was exhausted when I arrived home. I hit my bed; there is no greater comfort than sleeping in your own bed. I slept like a baby for a few days. My wife commented that I must really be tired because all I was doing was sleeping. I did not tell her about my ordeal; for all these years she has not known about these experiences until she reads this book.

When I was well rested she reminded me that I had not opened my mail. She disclosed that there was a letter from the lawyer.

I asked myself, "What did I do now?" I was a little under the weather and was not in the mood to open it. Finally, my wife took the letter and opened it; it was from the lawyer who had been trying to get in touch with me. I made the call. He wanted me to come to his Queen's Village office as soon as possible. A few days later I went down to his office and he informed me that the court matter had been finalized. Apparently the court found that the company was at fault for the injuries I had received and ordered the company to pay me quite a large sum of money. After all these years, the judge had finally ruled on the matter and made them pay for their mistakes and the suffering I went through. I actually thought that the case was finished because I gave up on it, but thankfully my lawyer did not. He pursued the matter until a decision had been made.

On hearing this news, the first thing that came into my mind was a promise I had made to myself during one of my spells at the hospital. I had undertaken to assist those who sought my help on health issues.

The lawyer handed me the check and said to me, "You are a good kid; you are too kind and they will eat you up out there." He also wished me the best of everything and a good life.

After I left his office, I thought about what he had said and realized that many persons with whom I had come into contact and who knew something about me told me would say, "You are a kind man" or "You are a good man." They all saw what I could not see. Sometime later on I heard that this gentleman, my attorney, had a stroke. I don't know whether he is still alive but for the time I interacted with him, he passed on some good advice to me.

Nineteen hundred and eighty-seven was a very interesting year. I was still working towards the goal of finding a cure. On Christmas day in nineteen hundred and eighty-seven, I was searching for a place to start a health food store because I thought I had enough knowledge of herbs gained from my parents and grandparents. I was familiar with what was healthy to drink and what was not. I also knew about good quality foods from growing up on a farm. I was also taught about the soil, so I felt that I had some tools to work with.

While driving on one of the country roads, I saw this sign, "Store for Rent." I went to a payphone and dialed the number. A gentleman answered me right away and promised to be at the location within half an hour. On his arrival, he introduced himself to me. I let him know what I was looking for. The price that was quoted seemed right at the time and so I went ahead and rented the place and started doing the necessary work on it.

The gentleman took a likeness in me and invited me to one of his other establishments some distance away. I will refer to him as Sam; he was of Jewish descent. We talked about some of the reasons I wanted to get into the health food business. I told him some of my "war" stories; he sympathized when he heard I had the sickle cell disease. He knew that this was a disease that ran in the children of Cush. I found out that he was one of the men who fought in the 1947 war when Israel captured the Golan Heights. He told me a lot about Israel and their struggles for independence and the fighting with their surrounding neighbors.

I worked diligently in order to get the store opened. It was a very difficult process then, starting up a business. There were so many legal documents to be signed; then the right products had to be sourced. I was able to open by the summer of 1988, although it was not a good time to open the store since most people were travelling on vacation. By then, also, I was already planning to depart on my next trip either in late September or early October and I had to find someone to manage the store while I was gone. I knew it was not a wise decision having recently opened a business, to leave it up to someone else who did not have the slightest idea about health, but I took the risk.

RETURNING TO TUCSON, ARIZONA

By late September 1988, I returned to Arizona to attend a Feast and to learn more. I stayed at the same hotel and the workers remembered me. They referred to me as the "rich gringo" because I was very generous with tips. I did not visit the desert museum on this occasion. I kept looking at the desert and its surrounding mountains from afar and I was extremely afraid of it. I respected it for its strict laws and harsh punishment. I kept my eyes opened to see if I would run into my "Angel" but I never laid eyes on her. I spent a lot of my time at the health food store.

One day I inquired of the attendant whether there was another health food store in the area and he said there was but it only sold products in bulk. He gave me the address and I took off anxiously to find it. It was like a warehouse and they carried bulk products. My greatest surprise was that they stocked some of the products I needed for the store such as: DeBoles Jerusalem Artichoke. I was also surprised that these products were manufactured in the New York metro, an area right in my neighborhood. One of the things I observed while I traveled around the country was that certain things led me right back to where I started and that was New York. It seemed as though the answer was right there in my backyard.

While in Arizona, I also tried to obtain information from the Native Americans who remained there, but they did not seem to know of the herbs that were used by their ancestors who roamed the west in earlier times. They were more into craft and the modern-day items that they sold to make a living.

I visited the museum in the city of Tucson where there was a lot of history on the walls in the museum and many antiques from their forefathers. Each tribe had their different symbols. I met a man named Jim who recently moved to the area. He invited me to his home where he lived with his wife; he did not have any children. I learned that his wife died a few years later. He took me around to quite a few places of interest. There were places I had not been to because I only heard of them just before I was about to leave. Some of those places included old Tucson, the City of Tombstone and Sonora. All those days I had been there no one mentioned these places until the night before I was about to leave.

Jim took some of us to John Wayne's Restaurant where representations of all his movies were displayed. The restaurant manager asked whether we had seen the sites mentioned earlier and we said, "No."

His response was, "If you have come this far and have not been to these places, then you have not been to Tucson. He also asked whether we had been to the Grand Canyon. I told him no, but the others had gone on that tour earlier in the week. Right then I considered returning to ensure that I covered every area. I thought that I had seen everything that I wanted to see but there was always something that I missed. I certainly did not want to miss anything.

One of the things I learned was that many bodybuilders both men and women who had contracts with companies would be there in the fall and winter working hard to get their pictures in the monthly body building magazines. The best sculpted bodies are usually featured in those magazines which flood the country on a monthly basis. I saw where those bodies are abused for a few dollars by the foods bodybuilders ate and drank at the hotel and other restaurants. The following morning they are in the gyms taking some sort of substance to get them going and when I see myself trying to fix mine and trying everything to overcome all odds, it hurt me to see what I saw that they could not see. I felt very sad.

As I looked around my hotel room and pondered on life from a different perspective, I asked the question, "Why me?" Why do some people go on in life without caring while others worry about the weather being too hot or too cold or what they will eat; they complained about everything in life. As I took walks towards the Civic Center on some of the hot days I would watch the little green lizards under the olive trees; when you got close to them they would run and hide and change their colors or they would run up the olive tree and blend in with the branches. I would linger a while and watch them and think about how wonderful life was. These creatures are usually in their environment living according to nature and they understand it quite well. Why can't we do the same? Why do we make life so complicated? We take our bodies given to us by the Creator, a superior being that gave us life and gave us the responsibility to be fruitful and replenish the earth, and destroy it before our days have come to an end.

I now know that after these forty plus years, all my health problems have come from what I consumed. I have grown to understand more about life and I know that I am what I eat and by eating all the wrong foods, the poisonous gas from the colon escaped into the blood which flows into the cells, got trapped in the T-cells which could not dispel the poisons. These cells have dispute between the white corpuscles and the red corpuscles. Since the white blood cells are greater than the red blood cells, the red blood cells cannot overcome the poisons; with the red blood cells not getting any of the elements that are required to nourish and tone them; the acid and the poison get into the joints and the rest of the sluggish organs; the liver works overtime to expel much of the poisonous waste stored in the lymph glands. When this occurs the body goes through tremendous trauma and most young persons do not survive this disease.

Remember, the human body has to work in harmony. It is the only way it knows how to function. The food we eat has to be in harmony so the minerals and enzymes have to be in perfect balance with the body; everything we eat has to be balanced. When the colon is out of balance, it means the colon is not getting the appropriate minerals for proper bowel function and rebuilding of the colon wall. The basic elements that are needed on a daily basis include: magnesium, sodium and potassium. Also, there is acidophilus for the colon lining to prevent plastic build up for the proper functioning of the colon. As I learned more about the colon and its role and function, I began to understand the nature of my problem and what was causing the numerous illnesses in mankind today. I suggest that the colon should be a more studied subject.

In nineteen hundred and ninety-five, I gave a lecture on colon management and the cause of diseases. A few persons walked out; they did not want to hear about their bowels because it was a private concern. However, those who remained commended me on the subject because they were all constipated and had not gone for a few days or, in some cases, weeks. By using over-the-counter laxatives and other stimulants, this caused damage to the bowel muscles, which in turn led to the poisoning of the organs.

Because of my chronic illness and the amount of medication I took, I, too, used to get constipated. I did not understand all these things at the time but by studying the colon and autopsies performed on colons and by noticing the body sculpture and shape I obtained sufficient knowledge to say that the body is lacking the proper foods and that the colon is starving from the lack of proper nutrients.

When autopsies are performed on the corpses of some movie stars and celebrities, the conclusion is usually there were problems with their colons. I did several studies on the colon and waste management and I found out that we eat three meals a day but we eat mostly unwholesome foods. It takes eighteen hours before that food is digested, enters the cecum and travels to the ascending colon then to the hepatic flexure, to the transverse colon, to the splenic flexure, down to the descending colon, to the sigmoid and to the rectum, where it enters the anus to be expelled. Approximately twenty-four hours of waste has built up in the five feet of the colon and cause all types of health problems; anything from cramps in our toes to heart disease or cancer; even the sickle cell that was poisoning me.

Illnesses are caused by eating devitalized foods. If the food is not whole or in its natural state or grown in the soil from which mankind came, then it should not be eaten under any circumstances. Many people seem not to understand the great gift of life. If we understood this body that was given to us, this beautiful temple to live in and enjoy, we would be a better people in all facets of life. The wisdom I have gathered from the Great I Am, grandparents and from what history has taught me and even some of the great ones who have gone ahead and left a tremendous amount of information for us today. After examining all the information I have come across and all that I have been through for the past forty-odd years, I have come to the conclusion that the colon is the most important organ in the human body; it is also the most neglected organ and the most abused organ in the human body.

I was not aware of how much I had to learn about my health, in general, until I began to examine the human body from a different perspective. I began to see things differently. I came to understand how to approach my health issues. One of the things I learned was to take control of my health because no one could do it better than me. I had a better understanding about the functioning of the organs and the importance of the right nourishment the body needs on a daily basis in order for it to function properly. I also observed that all diseases traveled the same route and then branched out because they start in the blood.

When I came to understand that life was in the blood; that changed everything for me. The body cannot heal itself properly if the blood is injured by poison or toxic chemicals. The blood has to be pure and clean for the body to operate at the speed of the energy force and the spark of life. When the foods we eat do not have the vital force from the elements we ingest, the mineral salts that become enzyme to clean buildup and energize the body; when these things are not taking place, the body will become sick; this is what happened to me. My body was not getting the minerals that formed the enzyme; my body was not getting its balanced amount and the blood was getting poisoned and this affected the weakest part. At that time, the blood cells could not fight back. They did not have the atoms, which were the missing link. The body requires sufficient enzymes to fight off diseases. I could go on and on to explain, but it will not do any good because you must understand the functioning of the body. I hope I have given you some kind of simple explanation.

A TRIP TO THE WEST COAST PALM SPRINGS, CALIFORNIA

While I was in Tucson, there were many conversations on health issues. I found out that persons in the west coast were more health conscious than any other persons I had come across and I said to myself, in the whole country someone somewhere has to be more involved than just a few so I became excited. I never thought much about Los Angeles. I always wanted to go where the air was cleaner but they suggested the desert. When that word "desert" came up, I ruled that out but it was explained to me that Los Angeles was like any major city with buildings, streets, pavements, hotels and everything that I could find in my city. Also, it was the home of famous movie stars. I understood that I could even walk on their footprints down town Palm Canyon Drive so I became enthusiastic about visiting Palm Springs.

In the nineties, I took my first trip to California in search of the cure for sickle cell anemia or anything that I could learn to help me in my struggle with this disease. Well, I headed for the west coast in the fall. When the announcement was made that we would be landing soon at the Los Angeles Airport, I kept looking out the window but I could not see the airport or the city. My first notion was that we would be landing in the water but I could not see any water either. It took a while for the plane to emerge from very thick smog and by that time, we were almost ready to land. That is how thick the smog was. It appeared as though the city was covered by this powerful force and when the plane burst through that thick fog, the hole closed up like nothing had been there before. This fog hung very low over the city. It caused me to start thinking that if this whole city was like this, then it could not be good for my health.

On landing, I proceeded to the car rental agency to obtain a vehicle to take me to my destination. When I arrived there it was like a circus because there were so many people seeking to rent a vehicle. Finally, after I informed them where I wanted to go and all the papers were filled out, I received a vehicle and was on my way. I headed east on the San Bernardino Freeway and within an hour, I was caught up in the most horrific traffic. Patience helped me to endure the stress. About nine o'clock that night I got into Palm Springs. I could not believe that I was actually seeing the stars in the dark blue sky. However, it was very hot. Upon asking a few questions I was able to find the Hilton, which was close to everything. My room was ready; everything was in order. I was too tired to eat after a long day driving in the heat. At that time of the year you would think it would be cooler but it was 105 degrees during the ten days I was there, so this weather was unusual for me because at that time of year I would be wearing warmer clothing.

I encountered many wealthy people holidaying there, some of whom I spoke to. I also made friends with the morning crew at the restaurant so that I could get fresh wholesome fruits for breakfast and lunch. They informed me there was a health food store half a block away from the hotel, right at the corner of Tahquitz and Palm Canyon Drive. I did not waste anytime getting there to see what they had in stock.

This health food store was called The Oasis, a very unusual name for a health food store. I got there some time during the day and introduced myself. I asked to see someone who was knowledgeable about the products, health and nutrition and was directed to a slim, tall, elderly silver-haired man, who I will refer to as Bill. My first impression was that he was vigorous, energized and walked with a spring in his step. I introduced myself and he asked whether I was from New York and I said, "Yes." He then informed me that he was from New Jersey but he had been in California for quite a while. I told him I was delighted to meet him. We walked back to the deli where they served juices, salads and meals. I ordered carrot juice and we sat and conversed for a while. He told me his story.

Apparently he left New Jersey in 1934 with seven dollars and walked to California and ended up in Hollywood. He got a job sweeping the streets; he then worked his way up and Dick

Powell, a famous Hollywood actor gave him a job. He saved enough and moved to Palm Springs. He also showed me a string of properties that he once owned. He believed that if he had kept those properties until the nineties, he would have been a multi-millionaire. He became a director of films and when Dick Powell died he worked with Howard Hughes directing movies. The last film he made was a movie called "Around the World in Eighty Days" in 1956. We spent hours talking, I had forgotten all about raising questions on health. During my time there he introduced me to many movie stars.

He used to say, "I want you to meet my friend from New York."

I shook the hands of so many interesting people during my travels. I met one of his sons, a fine kind man. Bill's wife had Alzheimer's disease so sometime during the day he would go to the house and look in on her. We shared many things; he was the one who told me about Essiac, a herbal tea formulated by a nurse, Rene Caisse. Apparently she had acquired the information from an old Indian woman before putting it to use. Bill also showed me the formula. As far as I know, I was one of the first to bring the formula to New York and the herbs to make it. There was a company in North Hollywood that had the right to distribute the herb when it was put together in its right formula. Bill was very knowledgeable in the use of vitamins; he told me he was only working to pass the time and to assist others with their health problems.

One day, I was introduced to the owner of the health food store. Bill informed her that I was also in the health field. Bill revealed that the owner's husband was a salesman, a very heavyset guy and so was his wife. He came upon the building, rented it and placed his wife there to run it. It was a way of keeping her from being bored. She, however, did not like healthy foods and hated the health business. This is how she found Bill who knew many people and with his background, it would be good for business. Her husband died from a heart attack and left her with the store and I understand that she was interested in selling it. I approached her about purchasing the business. I inquired about the price and was told $85,000. I promised to give her $20,000 in cash and the balance through the bank when I got back to New York. This was not in writing; just an oral agreement. However, after I returned home, I received a call from Bill that she was negotiating with a real estate agent. By the time I called her, she had already sold the property to someone who was in the real estate business, so I lost out on the deal. The store was in a prime location and was very profitable. I was thinking of moving to the west coast, but I guess it was not my time.

I returned to Palm Springs, CA several times and made quite a number of friends on those trips; I even took gifts for them on those visits. It was a place I liked. The new owner moved the store from the previous location to further up Sunshine Avenue and changed the name to

RX. It was a much larger building but not the same character or essence. It thrived in the new location but the new owner was not paying quarterly sales taxes. He wrote zero every quarter until the State caught on and held the owner and the business liable for all sales taxes. The Feds also had their people there each day to make sure that they got every cent the business owed for the years it had been cheating on both State and Federal taxes.

Well, the relationship between Bill and I grew. He wanted to return to his hometown and I offered to do everything I could to assist him. He gave me all the necessary information. I called the relevant body in New Jersey and provided them with all the information about the name of the town and all the rest of it. Even the Town Planning Board and City Hall were involved. When I received the report after months of searching, they indicated that the town no longer existed; they did not even remember the town. Well, when I gave Bill the news he was very disappointed; he really wanted to visit his old town in New Jersey to see what it looked like after all those years.

Bill was getting on in age and he was no longer needed at the store. Being at the store on a daily basis and meeting and talking with the customers meant everything to him. In 1995, Bill died of a stroke. The news of his death took something away from me. He was a mentor, a friend and somewhat of a father figure. I say this because we used to be alone in the store at ten o'clock at nights talking about health. However, if he had a greater knowledge about health, sickness and disease he would have been able to help his wife. Bill did not know then and I could not tell him because he has already left us. He helped so many persons whom he came into contact with over all those years while he was alive. Bill's teaching and guidance would continue on through others and me. The Essiac Herbal teas that others have used and the information that he passed on to me have ended up in the countries of Malta and Ireland where the Apostle Paul travelled in ancient times, where I understand, through a doctor, that cancer was a huge problem there and Essiac benefited many persons in that country with their health problems.

For many years I labored to find a means of extracting the juices from plants and fruits in their raw state until the fall of 1990 when I first met Bill. I inquired whether they had raw fresh juices and an attendant made me my first glass of raw carrot juice. It was like I was reborn having the first real life milk that comes from a mother's breast. While I was in Palm Springs, I spent most of my time at the health food store. I met a woman who grew wheatgrass and sold it to the store. She gave me a lot of information on wheatgrass, which she learned from Ann Wigmore, a holistic health practitioner and nutritionist. I also drank wheatgrass juice, it was the first time in my life that I was getting all the extra nutrients that the body needed. I also learned about a woman in the area who gave colonic irrigations. She had so many clients that she could not see me before I left. I was disappointed that I could not get at least one colonic irrigation before my departure but the few days I was there, I gathered a tremendous amount of information. The health food store was an information center for me. I also learned about how good Alfalfa sprout was for the body. All these must be consumed as fresh as possible.

One of the things that struck me as strange was that people would ask, "How is your colon this morning?"

I thought this was a very embarrassing question. It took me years before I really understood what this meant. It was the most health conscious place I had ever been.

Of course, there were those who were not interested in their health but the majority of persons I met were involved in some way. While I was there I did not participate in the nightlife, although there were many activities. It was a place where some of the world's wealthiest people lived and also a vacation paradise. Those things did not turn me on; I was there on a mission, so at nights I would be in my room reading books on health. I read books by Norma W. Walker, a pioneer in the field of vegetable juicing. Two of them are *Raw Vegetable Juices: What's Missing in your Body* and *Colon Health: The Key to a Vibrant Life*. Ann Wigmore also has a few books on Wheat Grass and on diet. There are many handbooks written about health. I spent my time learning the things that I needed to know. Palm Springs was truly a garden of knowledge for me.

I attended an October Festival while in Palm Springs. Vendors brought out their best products for sale on the main street, whether it was arts and crafts or other products. They would have the store's print on the sidewalk and all the fresh fruits: my favorite fruit was papaya. I had it every morning. I was there at the time that Lucy Arnez' print was placed on the sidewalk. Also on display were some rare books and other beautiful Native American beads and traditional blankets. There was so much to enjoy there in the desert that if I had to list everything it would take up too much space and time.

Many years ago I watched the movie "Palm Springs Weekend." A beach would be shown on the screen. When I got there I inquired about the beach and was told that it was several miles away. There was, however, a place called Oasis Water Park, which was a delightful place for a family day. There was a large area with water that could accommodate several persons at a time; the water made waves like one would experience on a beach. There was some kind of machine that stirred the water up like waves. I visited one day and there were many families having a wonderful time. There were also tram rides that went up over eight thousand feet to the mountain. My stay in Palm Springs, California was very fruitful and enjoyable but the time was up for me to return to the real world.

I returned to New York, rested up and reviewed what I had gained: knowledge, wisdom and understanding and this was what I have, the grace of the Great I Am. All these trips that I took around the country were for the purpose of meeting all those wonderful people and acquiring knowledge about my health. I also learned that it was not just about my health problem. I had to learn compassion, faith and humility because all the roads led me back to where I started. I had to learn about man's temple, that the body is the temple of the Great I Am where He would like to dwell but the body has to be clean—body, mind and spirit. It was not just about eating clean food that keeps the body healthy. It is what goes into the body as a whole. If the food is not good it would defile the body and then the structure would begin to shake or weaken and then you have to check to see whether it is spiritual, mental or physical because the human body must be in perfect harmony with itself. I have learned a great deal about the body over all these years.

In 1999, I had the opportunity to be a guest at the Whitaker Health Institute in Newport Beach, California. It was a new experience for me because it was the second time in my life that I was around a famous doctor who was known worldwide for his service to a new approach to health away from the modern-day medicine. The Health Institute deals with heart disease, diabetes, high blood pressure and some of the other common ailments. They also performed chelation therapy. I was there to experience how it was done firsthand. The patient would go to the hotel where the food was prepared; the food was selected each day for the patients. Those who were diabetic were given a different type of food. Foods were prepared for the patients based on their particular ailments. I noticed, however, that hydro-colon therapy and deep cleansing were not practiced. As I continued to read, I learned that when you neglect the colon you neglect life itself. For the nine days I spent there I learned quite a lot. There was a juice bar not too far from away, which I frequented to get a 16-ounce glass of carrot juice. I enjoyed this drink immensely. I was also fortunate to give table topics on health. I acquired a wealth of knowledge about people and their health. It took me years to understand why people could not see the same things or understand their health problems the same way that I did. When I talked to people they would say, "I got it from my parents" or "It's in the family genes" or "I don't know why God allowed this to happen to me." It was always a case of assigning blame elsewhere.

Yes, God made the blind, the deaf and the lame for a reason but He did not cause you to shorten your life by eating all those despicable, disease-carrying foods each day of your life, and when things start going wrong you quickly blame Him for your problems. He gave us laws and statutes to live by but we reject them each day because we allow man to teach us his way. Man's way leads to nothing but death before our time.

According to the Good Book, the way of a man seems right but the end thereof is always death.

My mother always inspired me with her letters of encouragement through my illness. In one of her letters she wrote, "What is man that the Great I Am or Jehovah or Yahweh was so mindful of?" It took me years to understand that God is love; God is a family. He is trying His best to bring mankind into His love and the only way that could happen is if mankind understands God's love because His love is the fulfilling of His laws. When we break these laws, they always break us. Well, my mother is no longer here but her words and her writings are still with me and echo in my heart. My mother, Dora Elizabeth, died in December 2005, one month before her ninety-six birthday. She left me a legacy of immense knowledge to take me through the rest of time.

There is no special magic in attaining and maintaining health. Whatever formula you may be given by anyone, if the entire body is not cleansed, it will not work. There are seven major organs that you have to pay great attention to by cleansing. Multiply the number of organs by seven times and that will give you the forty-nine cleansing of these lymph glands and organs that is necessary. Bear in mind always that life is the blood. Therefore, if the blood is not right, life will be extinct. If all the experts in the health field and those who have all these degrees in health understood how the human body functions, they would not use the amount of drugs and experiment by cutting the organs and believe that these practices will restore life to its fullest.

The Great I Am, The Great Jehovah and the Great Yahweh said, "Do not cut open the body or put any marks upon the body because you are a holy people unto me." We take for granted that we can consume anything and think it is fine. He said, "You are a holy people." That means you are special, very special so every thing we do with the body should be special.

I was speaking of the body and the forty-nine cleansing of the organs and the tissues. These are the seven major glands and tissues. First, there is the liver; all processes have to go through the liver for it is the machine of the body; the kidney is one of the liquid-waste dispensers of the body; the skin cells are also one of the major cells so that the sweat glands can perform its duty and prevent the pores from getting clogged; the lymph glands keep waste moving out of the body; the lungs are responsible for bringing in oxygen into the body and eliminating the carbon dioxide from the body; the bile has a major job to perform. It is responsible for the proper fluid that the liver is removing so that the juices can flow so that no calcium clots block the passage of the bile ducts. The colon is the greatest and most important organ of the body. There is no greater organ in the human body than the colon; it has a unique style in how it functions. The transverse colon moves from right to left and this boggles the minds of all the medical experts.

We are responsible for our own wellbeing, yet we hand over our bodies to the experts to manage them. So when we get sick they give us pills and when the pills don't work they would say, "We have to operate" and then the problem worsens. The organs which are already weak have no energy to support their functions, and are weakened further; then the body goes into trauma and cannot restore itself so what happens? Death is at the door.

I want you to take a look at this book. Take a look at the author, find out who is this man. I am the same yesterday, today and tomorrow if the Great One, Jehovah, permits it. For over twenty years I fought to understand this sickle cell trait or "sick cell" disease, as I refer to it. I was given up for dead. I searched the land for answers; I spoke to experts in the field; I have been in and out of hospitals for over 20 years and the answer I got was time; the time I had to invest in order to learn. That was the essence to my life. Not until I sought the Great I Am for answers—as my Mom said, "What is man that God is so mindful of?"

Yes, He was mindful of me. Because of His wisdom, His mercy and His love I am still alive today to say to you that all diseases can be overcome if you put your faith, your trust and your understanding in Him. He will give you the knowledge that you need to overcome the perils that are ahead of you. You have to get up; you have to work; you have to invest in yourself in order to get results. I have been through pain and suffering; I have traveled throughout most of this country searching for answers for my health. No one had the answer for sickle cell or sickle cell trait. Some people still don't know what it is. I had to travel to gain wisdom and understanding. I always had the answer but my mind was closed until the appointed time came for me to know.

For fourteen years, I fasted one to three times per month. During the fast, I would go without food and water. For thirty years, I ate raw salads; for thirty years I drank only distilled water. Change is an important feature of life; it is taking place around us constantly. If you are ill and you are unwilling to make changes to your daily living you won't survive because change is the required ingredient for overcoming. If you let deadbeat friends and family and your doctor fill your heads with deadbeat conversations, you will be in the same deadbeat sewer with the rest of them. Try to get out of your current condition otherwise you will be fighting a losing battle.

NEGLECTING THE COLON: A GREAT MISTAKE

I have had several colon therapies. In one year I have about forty-eight. Colon therapy is a must. The colon needs special nutrients at all times. Food must exit the colon within eight hours. Remember that it is the gas from the colon that is poisoning the blood. There are over three hundred poisonous gases in the colon, which the body has to fight off, especially if the food eaten is dead, and the colon's acidophilus pH is only fifteen percent and the billicus pH is eighty percent. The colon acidophilus pH should be eighty percent and the billicus pH should be fifteen percent. To obtain the proper balance, you should have several colonic therapies per year and an enema every night and morning. This is very important because the walls of the colon need three minerals: potassium, magnesium and sodium.

Clabber butter or matos is known in different parts of the world but in North America it is known as Kefer. It comes in different flavors. I recommend the plain favor because the other flavors may have too much sugar or acidophil or probiotics. You need to find a good brand. Food should be of the highest quality. Bear in mind that health has become a business and every expert who is involved in health will sell you anything and tell you that it is of high quality. If you do not understand food, then you will always be in trouble when you go shopping.

If you have a health problem and you are trying to restore your health then you must take these things seriously. Keep in mind that the greatest gift that we have is life. Without health you have nothing; everything you do depends on your health and, therefore, what you consume should be of value to you. You should be looking for quality foods and ninety-five per cent of the foods and juices you consume during the course of the day should be raw. Cooked foods serve the body no useful purpose. They in fact create all the problems you acquire each day. Flour should be avoided and also some grains, some nuts and some seeds. Remember that "organic" does not mean that the food is organic. There are certified organic what is organic has to do with the soil. It takes about twenty years with no interruption in the soil and no chemical use for the soil to be considered organic. Egypt was one of the world's richest organic areas. In Upper Egypt there is a process where the mountain moves and the water washes down the soil from the mountain; two bodies of water meet: the blue water and the white water rich in minerals and nutrients. It ends in the Africa's largest lake called the Queen Victoria Lake.

One of the nutrients that should be abundant in food is selenium. Our soil in the United States has been depleted from all its minerals and nutrients. Our soil is so poor that you can taste it in the food. Food could either mean life or death. If you eat the dead food you are just sustaining life; if you eat the right food you will have life and have it abundantly. Therefore, eating the right food is important. Vegetables of all kinds should be eaten; all the green leafy vegetables, kale, spinach, celery, broccoli, cucumber, collard greens, Swiss chards, peppers of all colors, romaine lettuce, green leaf, red leaf, dandelion, alfalfa, red and green cabbage, carrots, cauliflower, beans, asparagus and Brussels sprouts.

Carrots and lemons are two of the greatest foods on this planet. When you use them in their right state, they cleanse and rebuild the body.

Avocado, the natural fat that is so underrated is also food. It has beneficial fat to produce the right type of heat for the functioning of the glands. All these foods can be combined in whatever style that you chose. If you cannot eat them because the body is in a weakened state, they can be juiced or pureed.

Garlic is an antibiotic for the body. Two large cloves a day should be added to meals. It is one of the only raw nutrients that could get into the tissues, the glands and cells to remove all the waste that has been stored for years and the dead cells that are becoming parasites. Allicin, the nutrient in the garlic helps to open the gland tissues so the poisons can be removed through the sweat glands.

Herbal teas are very useful in any health problems. They can be beneficial in washing the body cells and organs with their unique style of operation. Pau D'Arco otherwise known as Taheebo is a South American herb which is very effective to clean the blood of fungus, fat, toxic chemical and other unwanted agents that affect the blood. Two to four capsules or three cups of strong tea steeped for twenty minutes should be taken daily.

Red clover is a blood purifier. Sage, violet, yellow dock, burdock and dandelion can be combined together or used separately.

Golden Seal is a very powerful herb and should not be used for more than seven-day cycles in small amounts. It has quite a stunning effect on the body. Remember, as I mentioned earlier, life is the blood so the idea is to do every thing that the body requires and to give it all the right nutrients that is necessary to maintain a healthy body.

Coffee and black teas have damaging effects on the body. They are the worst things used for enemas. As I learn more about their effects I move further and further away from them. The chemicals that they contain affect the heart muscle that pumps the blood to the arteries. These chemicals also interfere with the brain neutrons and result in mood behavior and place too much stress on the kidneys. They also act as bleach in the colon and remove the mineral salt from the colon and they also cause sluggishness of the liver. Although they have been widely used in clinics in North America for enemas, I recommend that they should not be used in any circumstances. Lemons can be effectively used instead. Also herbal teas, castor oil, spring water or plain water could be used for that purpose.

Likewise, Lewis Lab Brewers Yeast one or two tablespoons Heintzman's Farms golden flaxseed should be used daily three to five tablespoons of the golden flaxseed and lecithin two spoonfuls; one tablespoon of bee pollen granules on one or two slices of banana with some almonds, apricots, raw pumpkin seeds, raw sunflower seeds should be ground in a coffee grinder and eaten for breakfast. Nuts and seeds could become rancid because of their oil content and should only be prepared when ready to eat.

It is better for foods to be prepared fresh daily. If this is not possible, then food should not be stored in the refrigerator for more than three days. The body cannot use stale or spoiled foods, as it will ferment in the digestive tract before it gets to the stomach.

Mint teas are good for washing out the stomach.

Do not drink any milk unless it is fresh goats' milk and it should not be cooked. It should be taken warm for the stomach because of its tremendous benefit to the stomach lining and to prevent stomach ulceration.

Wheatgrass juice, which is chlorophyll, alfalfa juice, or barley juices are items that should be included in one's diet on a daily basis. Four to six ounces should be taken per day. They contain great nutrients for purifying the blood and improving the blood platelets. Remember organic foods and vegetables not only cleanse the system, they also nourish the body. Herbs are the cleansers, toners and strengtheners of the body and the raw foods are the proper roughage or the fiber and the gem of the body. The minerals, enzymes and the atoms are the energy force of life that produce energy; that is the spark of life found in the blood that causes us to live and that great life force in the hands of that Great Creator who once said, "Let us make mankind in our own image and likeness."

I have come a long way in these forty years and fought off all the odds to give you some insights that Jehovah has given me. Love is the stable pole; it is only love that can bring you through all difficulties. Through the years, I have seen the occurrence of a number of premature deaths, which could be attributed to either the dissemination of incorrect information or ineffective treatment as a result of lack of knowledge.

We are already living in a preexistent state because of what we are eating. The soft foods that we are eating have caused more harm to the human body than any population that is in the air. Look at all the diseases that are afflicting and killing the human beings prematurely today. We are given three score and ten years to live but by reason of the way we live, it will be four scores. Is anything in this universe greater than life? No, nothing matches the life that has been given to you so why don't you spend the rest of your days taking care of your bodies so that you could enjoy life and enjoy it more abundantly.

SICKLE CELL AND ITS TRAIT

Well, what is sickle cell anemia or sickle cell trait? They do have the same pattern. My version of this disease is simply that the white blood cells interact with the red blood cells. The white blood cells are throwing off their poisons into the red blood cells, which cannot overcome these poisons; the red blood cells cannot cleanse themselves in time to overcome the poison. This is only my version of sickle cell anemia or sickle cell trait.

The expert version is that sickle cell anemia is caused by a change in the chemical composition of hemoglobin which transports the oxygen inside of the red blood cells. Normal hemoglobin is a round ball-shaped folded molecule composed of forty protein subunits, two alpha chains and two beta chains. The chemical change is a valine amino acid substituted for glutamic acid in both of the beta chains. These chemical changes in hemoglobin cause the shape of the molecule to change under certain conditions such as lowered oxygen concentration and dehydration. Deoxygenated HG molecules can chemically link to each other creating these abnormal elongated hemoglobin polymer structures and distort the shape of the whole red blood cells. The abnormal red blood cells can damage the vessels around them and also the tissues that depend on the vessels for oxygen and nourishment. For example, the damaged red blood cells can cause thrombosis.

MOTIVATION IS THE KEY

Now that you have read what the experts have said about sickle cell and its traits and also my two cents about the disease, what are you going to do about your condition? I know you will go to the expert and get all the answers and then you will go home and do nothing because nothing inspires you because you lack the motivation to do anything. I must tell you that motivation is the key to success. I stated earlier that when I was a child, it was said that only poor people died when they were sick because they did not have the money to pay the doctors and I believed this until 1957 when I learned about this wealthy man who was ill and hired one of the best doctors from Oxford University, London to treat him, but died nonetheless. Although the doctor tried everything that medical science offered but he could not save this man's life.

Now, this man had all the wealth in his possession and yet all his wealth could not save him. It took years for me to understand that all flesh will die but life is a gift that you do not abuse. Life is like a gem that you nourish and feed until Our Father says it is time. In my case, this was the motivation to make me rise to the occasion. It takes motivation to achieve any goal.

When I was a boy my grandparents used to wake me up at four o'clock in the morning to go to the fields. They never used a timepiece to wake them. Today, everyone I know has a clock; some even have more than one in each room, set to alarm at different times to get them out of bed. This is their motivation. Despite this, however, many times they are late or never get to their destinations because the alarm clocks lost time. The story of the prophet Moses moves me because it took great courage and motivation to stir him to go up on the mountain where The Great I Am dwelt at that time, to ask him that question, "Why?"

Let no one tell you what you can or cannot do. There are many books out there to inspire and educate. Knowledge is power. *The Seven Laws of Success*, for instance, teaches you all these things. One of the seven laws is health, which is the most important one because if you are not healthy, then your life is diminished. So my advice to you is to take charge of your life. As the Creator once said, "Today, I have given you life and death, you choose."

The human body is a temple. Mankind was designed, as we were told, by organic matter, the highest quality of the ingredient matter. He breathed life into the nostril of man and man became a living soul. Next, we were told that the Great Jehovah planted a garden East of Eden. Why did Jehovah plant a garden? Why did

He not tell man, "You have enough flesh here, kill and eat?" It is because He knew that flesh rots and dies. Also, because man was made in His image, man has to be of a high quality; His Temple has to be of superior condition.

The human body is made up of over fifty trillion cells: t-cells, b-cells, k-cells and so on. All of them should be in harmony with each other and to keep all these cells in harmony they require to be bathed constantly in an enriched environment. These trillions of cells are fed by the nutrients that we put into our bodies on a daily basis. The blood has to be purified and kept clean so that life could remain intact until The Great God of this Universe takes it away in its due time. This body depends on all many nutritive elements that are required to maintain, rebuild and clean the entire system, and these elements must come from the richest organic soil if we are to benefit. If these elements are not rich in nutrients then illness and early death will occur.

One of the greatest nutrients in the soil is selenium. Most of our North American soil is depleted of this rich nutrient. If the human body does not obtain enough selenium, an agent called free radicals takes over the body and become a doorway for diseases to enter the body—anything from joint pains, heart disease, kidney failure, stroke, liver damage, cancer and a whole host of other ailments. Therefore, the soil in which the food is grown is extremely important.

In the Upper Nile Valley, Egypt, there is a process that has been going on since the beginning of time where the silt, mud and the vegetation are washed down from the mountain by two rivers called the White Nile and the Blue Nile. When those two waters join together with the rich nutrients that enrich the soil, then the foods grown in this soil are rich in the elements. If the soil has no life, then the food is dead. So by eating dead food the body becomes dead, making us a pre-existing life, not a vibrant life that is full of energy; just existing from day to day.

In 1936, the Agriculture Department was informed about the soil depletion and advised to make some effort to restore it. However, that warning was ignored. It is my view that the poor soil is one factor contributing to the high incidence of many diseases and health woes affecting us today.

A few years ago, I underwent surgery on my shoulder and when the surgery was over and the drugs wore off, I experienced tremendous pain on my upper body and was prescribed painkillers. I, however, refused to take them. The nurse informed me that if I did not take them my blood pressure would rise and I could have a stroke.

I said to her, "I know what pain is like. You don't have pain until you have sickle cell disease."

It could be one of the most deadly diseases when the body is starving for oxygen. Oxygen is the greatest neutralizer for the body. When there is a lack of oxygen the tissues are swollen and they block the flow of oxygen from doing its job. The iron in the blood pushes the oxygen through the body and as long as there is any type of inflammation in the body there will be pain. When the body is sick, the body will become inflamed—a sign of illness somewhere.

When you are experiencing pain as a result of sickle cell, that pain is coming from deep inside the blood so that even the bones in the body ache. If the blood does not have enough oxygen to do its job and as long as the body does not have sufficient oxygen we will always suffer the great agony of having to deal with pain. The blood has to be always in peak shape to efficiently supply these trillions of cells. If the blood is unhealthy, we would continue to have suffer health issues such as sickle cell and other degenerative diseases.

I have given you quite a bit of information about this disease that affects some people in particular. As every race on this earth has some kind of disease that affects them, all one has to do is to look at one's family's eating history and if you look long and hard you will find the answer there. If you look at the food that this race ate for a hundred years to this present day you will know why sickle cell is a great concern in our people who have poor understanding about this disease.

I hope that this book will open the eyes of those who have read it to understand that there is another way to approach this disease that deforms babies, children and even grown-ups.

You have read about this man who has triumphed over this deadly disease. I was once told that a doctor has to teach his patient everything he knows but the physician is the one to treats the patient. Well, I have provided you enough information about my experience and knowledge of sickle cell and sickle cell trait and I hope this book will make a difference in your life.

I am the subject of this book. If I did not think the information provided was beneficial to you, I would not have recorded it. I know because I have survived for over thirty years since given the death sentence of "five more years to live."

My strategy over the last twenty years of struggle with this disease focused on the food and water I consumed, special baths and exercise. These are some of the vegetables I have used throughout the years. All of them could be eaten raw or juiced.

1. Vegetables

Green leaf lettuce	Parsley
Romaine lettuce	Spinach Leaves
Red leaf lettuce	Collard greens
Celery	Radish
Kale	Cauliflower
Cabbage (green, red)	Broccoli
Shitake Mushroom	Tomatoes
Peppers (Green, Orange, Red, Yellow)	Sprouts and their seeds
Garlic (White, Red)	Brussels sprouts
Onions (Red, Yellow	Alfalfa sprouts
Avocado	Sunflower sprouts
Beet	Bean sprouts mix
	Wheatgrass juice and some of the other sprouts

2. Water

Water is very important. One of the best drinking water is the Mountain Valley Spring Water. Two to three 10-ounce glasses of water should be had on a daily basis. Also, a pint of distilled water should be taken each day. The brain needs tremendous amounts of nutrients to function effectively. It is part of the nervous system that involves the spinal cord. The brain requires mineral salts in their natural form. Distilled water soothes the brain. Find a good source of water in whatever city you live.

3. Baths

Baths are also vital to help the cells when they are exhausted from overwork due to the toxins in the body. Take baths with four pounds of Epsom salt in the water three times per week.

4. Exercise

Exercise is another very essential aspect of healthy living. The limbs and the bone structure are badly abused and exercise strengthens and repairs the bone.

There are many books out there on sickle cell anemia and sickle cell trait. You can find lots of valuable information at any library around the country or you may call any State Department of Health who could provide you with enough information on this disease. Every hospital in the country has some method for treating this disease such as bone marrow transplant, blood transfusion, painkillers and a host of other treatments that are far advanced than previously. If you write to:

Howard University
2121 Georgia Avenue, NW
Washington, DC 20059

or call 1-202-865-8292, they would send you information on sickle cell and its traits.

I hope I have provided you enough information to help you manage this deadly disease. I close with love.

ACKNOWLEDGEMENTS

I sincerely thank Mrs. Linda Mondesire for inspiring me to write this book. It was at the worst time of my life when I was at the lowest ebb of my life with the death of my son, she said to me, "You need to write that book." She said, "No words could soothe your pain but writing your story will help you overcome some of the pain in life that you would have to go through."

I also thank my loving wife Denise Sandy for supplying me with some of the materials that I needed to write this book. Also for your support and space she afforded me to write.

I say a special thanks to a special lady, Tammy Lewis, who was my rock, and who encouraged me each day. Even when I was bruised with pain and wanted to give up, she spurred me on; she was my encourager. One afternoon she saw me struggling with an eraser and sharpener and she asked, "What are you doing?" I said, "I am working these erasers." She promised she would be right back. She returned with some improved writing tools that made the job easier. She saved me a lot of frustration. I really appreciate her wisdom and thoughtfulness.

I also thank all of my friends who offered words of encouragement when they found out that I was writing this book.

In my lifetime, I have been in the presence of some notable people, like Haile Selassie I of Ethiopia and I even had the pleasure to meet and shake hands the Queen of England, governors at the U.S. Capitol and senators. With all the great people I have encounter, by far the greatest is the Creator of the Universe. Although I have never seen Him or the Son, I know They are always with me. I do not have to guess. I could not have gained all this understanding, wisdom and knowledge without the Creator and His Son, Jesus Christ. Here I express my gratitude.

Most of all, I thank the Great I Am for strengthening me with His wisdom, granting me the patience and humility at a difficult time in my life. Without His compassion and His love and the love of Jesus Christ, it would not have been possible for me to accomplish this task at such a critical time of my life.

Last, but by no means least, I thank Ms. Jean Sandy who typed and performed a first edit of this book.

For further information please contact:
    Healthy Garden Health Center Inc.
    288 Ronkonkoma Avenue
    Ronkonkoma, NY 11779
    Phone: 631.471.3335
    Web: www.healthygardenhealthcenter.com
    Email: zeke@healthygardenhealthcenter.com

We are a health centre providing consultations, cleansing, juicing and raw foods to rebuild the body to its natural state.

ABOUT THE AUTHOR

Mr. Ezekiel Sandy is a highly trusted and brilliant community leader in the health care industry. Mr. Sandy has dedicated his life to the well being of others, both mind and body. He has made heart and health issues his personal responsibility. With over 40 years in the industry, his consulting abilities are sought worldwide.

Good health is a gift you can truly give yourself and famous nutritionist Mr. Zeke Sandy, President of The Healthy Garden Health Center, Inc. has had the opportunity to promote healthy eating, by lecturing and conducting seminars on healthy eating habits throughout the United States. During his tremendous journey, he has given much hope and inspiration to others on how to live a healthy life by eating nutritious foods.

In 1998, Mr. Sandy was a guest at the Whitaker Institute Medical Center in Newport Beach, California. The topic of discussion was about the advantages of Chelation Therapy and Mr. Sandy addressed the attendances with concerns pertaining to their own health issues. In 2003, Mr. Sandy prepared and presented a health seminar at Southold Town Recreation

Center in Peconic, New York and talked about his own miraculous healing from the use of natural herbal foods. In 2004, he was interviewed by the Long Island Business Newspaper at this store in Ronkonkoma, New York where he discussed good health and wellness results from including natural foods in your daily diet. In 2006, Mr. Sandy was a guest at the Long Island Holistic Medical Association monthly meeting where he met with a variety of medical practitioners to discuss the advantages of using herbal foods.

In February 2006, Mr. Sandy presented a weight loss seminar on healthy eating habits at Lamonico Restaurant in Centereach, NY. In April of the same year, he was guest speaker at Dowling College in Oakdale, NY where he lectured on the importance of choosing the rights foods that add nutritional balance for children who suffer from ADD, ADHD, PDD, and Sensory Dysfunction, and in June, he also lectured at P.T.C. Medical, P.C. in Patchogue, NY on the preparation of nutritious foods for special needs children. In 2009, The Healthy Garden Health Center, Inc. presented and conducted a lecture on diabetes and the types of healthy meals required to help combat and control this medical problem.

In 1988, Mr. Sandy opened his first health food store in Selden called Health & Nutrition. Two years later, he relocated to Coram opening King Solomon's Health Food Store. Need for expansion resulted in Mr. Sandy relocating once more. Ezekiel Sandy opened his store Healthy Garden Health Center in 2003, where he continues to consult clients on health and nutrition, as well as treating numerous clients around the world, through his extensive knowledge of using all natural products from the earth to treat and heal the human body.

05491681

CPSIA information can be obtained at www.ICGtesting.com
Printed in the USA
LVOW06s1510300514

387959LV00001B/51/P